HOUR 30

An Uncensored Memoir of a Doctor-in-Training

by

Brandon Musgrave, M.D.

Hour 30
Copyright © 2012, by Brandon Musgrave.
Cover photograph by Noel Kelley. Used by
permission.

For information about special discounts for bulk purchases, please
contact Sunbury Press, Inc. Wholesale Dept. at (717) 254-7274 or
orders@sunburypress.com.

To request one of our authors for speaking engagements or book
signings, please contact Sunbury Press, Inc. Publicity Dept. at
publicity@sunburypress.com.

FIRST SUNBURY PRESS EDITION
Printed in the United States of America
May 2012

Trade paperback ISBN: 978-1-62006-064-3
Mobipocket format (Kindle) ISBN: 978-1-62006-065-0
ePub format (Nook) ISBN: 978-1-62006-066-7

Published by:
Sunbury Press
Camp Hill, PA
www.sunburypress.com

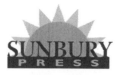

Camp Hill, Pennsylvania   USA

Acknowledgments

The process of writing a book during some of the most difficult years of my training was not an easy task. Furthermore, the work that goes into a book after it has been written is just as extensive. Without Sunbury Press, and owner Lawrence Knorr, this book would never have been possible. I would like to thank my editor, Allyson Gard, for her brilliant job at polishing 'Hour 30' to perfection. It is because of these two individuals that you are able to read this memoir.

There were also two amazing individuals that assisted me in crafting the final version of 'Hour 30' prior to submission to Sunbury Press. Mary Musgrave and Carol Patterson aided in bringing a rough draft to a more readied version. I will forever be thankful for their efforts.

The clever title of "Hour 30" was created over a dinner table at my sister-in-law's wedding. Special thanks to Jacob Hernandez for his creativity in choosing the title, which illustrates quite well the strength and stamina needed to succeed in medical training.

On a more personal note, I want to thank the many physicians and patients I worked with at Loyola. It is because of their openness in sharing their life with me that I took up writing.

Nicole, my wife, played an instrumental role in my professional development over the years. I thank her for having patience with me while I worked long shifts and spent many hours writing in coffee shops. Not all wives would be so supportive, and I wouldn't blame them, either. Thank you, Nicole, for believing in this important message.

Finally, I give thanks to God for making me who I am today, and who I will become in the future. I give thanks for the skills that He gave me to make a difference in the lives of many through surgery and medicine.

Table of Contents

Chapter 1: Introduction

As I walked past the patient in the adjacent room, I saw that she stared up at the ceiling with obvious nervousness. I had no idea at the time that she would be dead in half an hour.

When I got back to my room in the specials lab, the anesthesiologists were still trying to wake our aneurysm patient. My attending physician, or simply "attending", came back into the room to do another neurological exam.

"Ma'am, can you open your eyes?" the attending said.

No response.

"Ma'am!" he shouted.

No response.

He reached over to her shoulder and pinched her as hard as he could, his voice elevating dramatically.

"WAKE UP!" he shouted as he ripped off her oxygen mask and began smacking her in the face.

"This isn't normal," he said. The anesthesiologist agreed.

"INDUCE HER! WE'RE GOING BACK IN!"

The room went into a flurry of activity as they prepared to get into her vasculature. I helped as well as I could, injecting heparin into saline bags for the procedure. The attending moved faster than I had ever seen him move. We called for neurosurgery in case emergency surgery would be needed. When dye was injected into the brain, a large clot could be seen adjacent to the coil. The dye-filled portion of the artery had narrowed right behind the coil, signifying that the vessel lumen was full of clot. We began blasting her with clot-busting medicines in the artery, extremely dangerous medicines that can easily cause hemorrhaging in the brain. Hour after hour we fought to save her from stroking out and dying, recording each clot buster dose as we quickly approached the danger level.

It is bizarre how major events always seem to happen at once in the hospital. Right across the wall from our room, the code to resuscitate the patient I had seen earlier began. Both rooms were now in a panic to save their patients. It

1

was not a good day for the specials lab. Unfortunately, the other patient was not as fortunate as ours.

**

Matthew 25:36, "For I was ill and you cared for me."

These are the words that I strive to live by. My name is Brandon Musgrave, and I am a 2008 graduate of Loyola University Chicago Stritch School of Medicine. After medical school, I decided to perform a residency in the field of Otolaryngology- Head & Neck Surgery. This field is commonly referred to as Ear, Nose & Throat (ENT). Halfway through my third year of medical school, I realized that I had a story to tell.

Remarkably, during the first six months of writing, I had no idea I was writing a book. Through a need to share my experiences in my medical training, I actually began by posting journals online for my family and close friends to read. I had both good days and bad days, but I always felt blessed to be a part of such a wonderful medical school, with each day full of challenges, each one teaching me something invaluable. I must warn you that there are many parts of this book that are somewhat unpleasant in nature and may be difficult to read; however, I decided early on that, if I was going to write this book, I was not going to censor it.

The purpose of what you see before you is the telling of the story of an American medical student. Some details have been changed to protect the identities of the patients whose stories I will tell. These patients taught me more than I could ever have taught them about disease, suffering, and spirituality. I hope that you enjoy this book because I have poured myself into it; and, hopefully, once you are finished, you will have a better understanding of the grueling process that is medical school.

After high school, one must attain a bachelor's degree from a university in order to apply to medical school. It can be any degree you want as long as you fulfill the scientific requirements of each school to which you apply. Each year, the number of applicants increases, and medical schools have become more competitive. You must be at the top of your class, both in high school and college, to be a competitive medical school applicant. The standardized test, the MCAT, is taken during your junior year of college and takes about four months of preparation to be done properly. While I scored in the top ten percent nationwide with a nearly perfect GPA from the University of Illinois, I was still rejected from many medical schools.

This information is not meant to discourage any pre-medical students out there but, instead, to motivate, to "light a fire" under you, similar to what the many mentors I had in college did for me when I needed a little pushing. The process is definitely worthwhile... particularly when you receive your first acceptance letter. I was at Rush Medical School in Chicago for a conference when I received my first acceptance. I simply walked into the admissions office and asked whether or not I was accepted. An envelope was handed to me with my fate enclosed. Although I ended up choosing Loyola, it was a moment of remembrance that I won't easily forget.

Medical school is four years long with each year different in its own way. The first two years are the basic science years, consisting of classes with little patient contact. Think of it as college on steroids. During the first year, you learn everything you can about the human body, through anatomy and physiology. During the second year you learn everything that can go wrong with the body and the medications used in response. The last two years consist of rotations through the different medical specialties. The majority of this book will deal with the last two years of medical school and the patients I encountered during this time.

Everyone rotates through the same core specialties during third year, while fourth year is highly individualized for each medical student. These electives serve the purpose of preparing each student for his/her specific specialty. After all of this hard work, a medical degree is finally awarded. Unfortunately, this means little more than a license to begin residency, the specialization of doctors into the fields of their choice. It consists of the most grueling hours of the training process and the first time a professional student gets real responsibility.

This book will not discuss residency; instead, it addresses the process of medical school and the struggles faced on both a personal and professional level. I will take you with me on the journey I faced during these four challenging years of my life. The vast majority of this book is personal. It's about interesting patients I met that touched my life in a significant way. While some stories are sad, others are uplifting. Overall, I hope you take something away from this book that is more than a momentary emotion. I hope you learn to appreciate the unique bond formed between doctors and patients, especially a doctor-in-training. These patients were kind enough to invite me into their lives at their most vulnerable moments. My intention is to do them justice so that their memories will live on.

My interests in medicine were cultivated when I participated in a government internship program in the state capital of Springfield during my last semester of high school. Dressed in my first white coat at the tender age of eighteen, I was shadowing a cardiologist, daily experiencing the incredible "real world of medicine," while barely old enough to drive. For a time, I was the talk of St. John's Hospital and its associated clinic, Prairie Heart Institute. No one could fathom why a teenager was working hand-in-hand with a board-certified interventional cardiologist. As a result, I quickly acquired the nickname "Doogie."

During my time there, I saw patients, witnessed invasive procedures, and helped with basic office work, motivating me for the upcoming years of training. Numerous people warned me that I would have to bury my nose in books for ten to fifteen years if I really wanted the title of "MD" hanging behind my name. Something about their challenge excited me all the more as I headed off to the University of Illinois at Champaign/Urbana a summer early to begin classes.

My time at the "U of I" was very interesting. I studied so hard I barely had time to make friends or have fun. Luckily, I had a roommate who shared my ambition and even scolded me a few times when I began to slack a bit. The determination began to pay off as I often received the highest scores on my midterms in classes that sometimes numbered from 150-450 students. I say this not to brag but to remind my readers that there is much more to medical school admissions than grades.

I was accepted into only a few medical schools in the state of Illinois. Although I volunteered in an emergency department and a nursing home, I didn't put the passion into volunteering that I should have. I believe this played a part in some of my rejections. With so many applicants these days, medical schools have the luxury of choosing between the students with the grades as well as with the extra-curricular activities.

During my junior year at the U of I, I met the woman who would later become my wife. I mention her here because she brought me down to earth and taught me more than a textbook ever could have. Among these lessons is that life is about more than science and textbooks; it's about relationships and family. Acquiring these skills early on helped me to better realize what type of doctor I wanted to be. Being the most intelligent and talented doctor around is nothing if I can't relate to the patients I am treating. It bears repeating: life really is about relationships. Together Nicole and I decided in my senior year that I would attend Loyola University Chicago Stritch School of Medicine. Thus began some of the most difficult and exciting years of my life.

Chapter 2: The Basic Science Years

The first two years of medical school contain very little patient interaction. Loyola, along with many other schools nation-wide, is trying to change this by getting students into the hospital earlier. Still, the majority of time is spent in classes and private studying to master the basic sciences. My first semester focused on cell biology and anatomy, with nine grueling weeks in the anatomy lab in the basement of the medical school. I can still remember the pungent odor that nearly knocked me over when I first entered the lab. The long corridor leading to the cadaver crypt was lined with cross sections of real bodies for all to see, resembling something out of a cheap horror flick. Then I saw that each tiny piece of anatomy was labeled for the learning process. Inside the lab I noticed jars along the walls, containing dead, grossly-disfigured babies. Here was the opportunity, although unnerving, to bring to life the disfigurements and congenital abnormalities we read about in the textbooks.

We were separated into groups of four with our own cadaver to dissect. As we opened the body bag for the first time, I was surprised by the creature that lay before me, no longer looking human, the skin appearing more leather-like than the warm, soft skin we know. The formalin used to preserve the body was so pungent that we began to wonder which smell would be worse: the formalin or the smell of decaying flesh. It permeated our clothes and, despite using gloves, we could not get the smell off our hands. For weeks, every time I ate, I could still detect the odor when I brought my hand near my mouth. I still find it humorous when I am in an elevator with first-year medical students during the fall. They don't realize it at the time, but they smell like anatomy lab. In confined spaces, every senior medical student knows who the first-years are because we have all been through the process.

Many students had difficulty the first day with more than just the smell. I remember one classmate's statement that she couldn't sleep at all after the first night of dissection. Throughout the course, many groups kept a wet rag over the face of their "patients" in an attempt to subdue the too-personal experience of looking into their eyes while doing what seemed like the ultimate degradation.

We began the dissection on the patient's back. Surprisingly, we got little direction on how to proceed except for a quick lecture at the beginning of each day and a computer tutorial next to our cadaver cart. So, on that unforgettable day, we began stripping all of the skin off the backs of our cadavers. In order to retain the cadavers' moisture, we kept the large folds of skin in order to wrap up the skinned bodies at the end of the day's dissection. After we had identified and memorized every small muscle and tendon in the back, we began stripping them away to get to the vertebrae, or backbone.

After vigorously scraping the tiny muscles away, I distinctly remember thinking it looked like tuna. My colleague and I used a power saw to open the bones and thereby see the spinal cord. We took great care as we opened up the dura, the delicate covering of the cord, in order to preserve the anatomy.

The arms were next and were unexpectedly difficult. An amazing number of nerves, arteries, and muscles in the arm branch and diverge to provide the delicate movements of our fingers. We had to know every branch, every muscle, everything. We placed the "de-gloved" skin from the arms at the cadaver's feet, again using it for moisture retention at the end of each day. Those students who did not follow this daily ritual ended the nine weeks with dried body parts that were very difficult to use.

After the arms, we proceeded diligently to the head and neck, by far the most difficult and challenging structures of the human body. The brain, however, was saved for later. Before we even started, the instructors removed the brains for purpose of dissection in the second-year medical students' neuroscience class. They were returned to their rightful bodies for cremation at the end of the course.

7

This was the point where the class became more difficult. In order to learn the treacherous domain of the deep face and sinus cavities, we used a large saw to cut the face down the middle. Approaching a perpendicular angle, we then cut the skull in half from the side. We ended up with a quartered head with the needed cross sections to see the tiny nerves and arteries hiding deep within the recesses of the skull. Every curve, notch, and fissure in the skull had to be identified and memorized. We placed the two front quarters on the cadaver's chest with the attached pieces of neck. For days on end, we carefully and meticulously dissected through each and every square centimeter.

We had an anatomy book at the head of the table and referred to it every few minutes to make sure we were studying the right structure at the right time. After uncovering a new or before-unseen nerve or artery, we would say the name multiple times out loud to lock it into our memory banks. Although I had not made my decision at this point to pursue ENT, I should have seen the writing on the wall. Interestingly enough, the only time I ever scored the highest on an exam in my class in medical school was on the head and neck exam. I am confident that this rigorous and formative training will assist me during my training in and practice as an ENT.

The thorax and abdominal cavities were next on the list. Although the anatomy is very interesting and unique, we progressed very quickly because the organs are large and easy to learn. In fact, I don't think we took more than a day or two on the entire chest cavity. My particular cadaver had died of esophageal, or throat cancer, pathology we were particularly interested in seeing up close. When we had finally made our way to the esophagus, we found a grotesque tumor, a mass of greenish-black chunks obliterating the normal tissue. Curious, we began walking around to the other cadavers to observe other interesting findings. One in particular stands out above the rest. He had a penile implant, which seemed to amuse most of my class. The professors admitted that this was actually a common finding. After the fun was over, we returned to the work at hand.

The pelvis was much more difficult to learn than anticipated. For one thing, all of the anatomy seems to dive into this abyss that is the pelvic floor. In addition, the nerves and arteries branch into this cosmic puzzle with which I am still uncomfortable. In order to proceed with some accuracy, we once again had to break out the saw. We quartered the pelvis, cutting off one entire leg with half the pelvis still attached. Just as in the deep face, the views we needed had to be exposed. My group was the first to get to this step in the process; while my colleague sawed and severed the section, I pulled it, receiving a number of stares and gasps as I nearly tumbled backwards with a leg in my hands. I must admit, it was a funny feeling holding a human leg. I remember joking that only two types of people ever do something like this: medical students and serial killers. After we had finished dissecting the legs, similar to the arms, the whole process was over.

The final exam took place right before Christmas. We had one minute per station, where the instructors had placed one to two numbered tags on each corpse, totaling over seventy tags, including a few on the model skeletons. We walked from cadaver to cadaver, room to room, in silence. The whole process is like an induction ceremony of sorts, a rite of passage. You are officially a medical student when you go through the macabre but necessary process of gross anatomy lab. After we finished that year, we gathered downstairs for a ceremony of thanks and remembrance for the generous souls who donated their bodies to science. When asked if we would donate our bodies after going through the course, we all shuddered at the question, which goes to show that it takes an amazing person to give such a gift to humanity. It is certainly better for medical students to learn anatomy for the first time on deceased individuals than on the operating table with live patients.

After anatomy, school returned to the more mundane way of learning, using classrooms and textbooks. The structure of the first two years centers on lecture and small groups. Generally speaking, the morning has two to three lectures followed by a small group session or a lab. The recent trend is to have really short days and more time for self-study. I thought this was great because I learn much better on my own than in a lecture. Sometimes the days were as short as a few hours, while others would last all day. This problem-based learning works only if students are willing to use their newfound free time to study and not squander it. It becomes apparent who did what when board scores arrive.

Small group sessions were broken into groups of five or six students with a physician facilitator. Under the guidance of a doctor, we discussed case studies about patients with specific diseases covered that day in lecture. Because lecture sometimes lends itself to lull students to sleep, the group study approach is a great way to learn since you are actively applying the knowledge presented in lecture. The combination of pre-lecture study, lecture itself, and application of this knowledge is a triple punch, allowing you to review the material three times in a twenty-four-hour period. It becomes strongly ingrained at this point even though, of course, it has to be reviewed once again the week before the test. Labs outside of gross anatomy and neuroscience consist of mostly computer-based pathology slides, which have made the microscope obsolete. The slides are now uploaded onto software programs so students can focus their time on memorizing what cancer cells look like instead of flipping through decaying slides. Within the last couple of decades the learning base for medical knowledge has broadened, thus requiring the medical student to absorb a vast amount of information to achieve medical expertise. For this reason, instructors have to find ways to become extra-efficient and increase the learning curve per teaching session.

Second semester of first year consisted of physiology and host defense, wrapping up our study of normal human anatomy and function. I had a few months' break after first year in which I participated in cardiovascular research, a small project about aortic aneurysms. One interesting part of the project is that, although I didn't get a great turnout in terms of patient participation, I did save my first life. This was a patient who, on follow-up CT scan, showed a very large aneurysm that risked rupturing at any moment. Upon notification, he elected for immediate surgery and had it grafted to prevent further dilation. A couple more patients had surgery before the project was over; many more were found to have smaller aneurysms and are being closely followed. I don't think I will ever forget the moment of saving my first life. It didn't matter that I had never met the patient. I was beginning to experience some of the fulfillment of why I went into medicine in the first place.

My second year began with neuroscience and pharmacology. Learning about the brain with all of its complexity was a formidable task. The course combined both anatomy and pathology, so we learned about the nerve pathways through the brain and which disease presented upon their injury. In a few weeks, we had learned all of the nerves in the body and their course of travel. For instance, a pain pathway from a fingertip makes its way to the spinal cord, criss-crosses to the other side, and then travels up to the brain. Also, different types of nerves serve each type of sensation: pain, vibration, light touch, deep touch, and position sense. This doesn't even include the motor nerves that control every muscle in the body, as well as sweat glands, salivary glands, and the pupils in the eyes.

Everything was fair game for the exam. I found the class a bit overwhelming and much more difficult than first year. Some of the pathology seen in neurology, however, is quite intriguing. Even though, anatomically, the two halves of the brains look similar, each side is dominant over the other in different aspects. The left side, in most individuals, is dominant for speech. The right, on the other hand, is used more for association and thinking.

Reported cases of patients who have had either trauma or stroke in the right side of the brain subsequently cannot comprehend "left." Remember, the nerves often criss-cross to the opposite side of the brain. Give this stroke victim a razor and he will shave only the right side of his face. Give him a plate of food and he will eat only the right half. Have him copy a picture of a clock and he will only draw 12 to 6. In fact, if you were to grab the left hand of one of these patients and show it to him, he will tell you it is your hand. Luckily, this bizarre phenomenon is usually temporary. Patients will slowly recover what was lost if the damage to their brains wasn't permanent. I remember describing this disorder to my family over dinner at a restaurant and looking up to see the entire table next to us listening intently. It is perhaps the most puzzling phenomenon I have learned about to date.

Every so often one of the famous neurosurgeons at Loyola would come and give a clinical lecture. As medical students, we loved a good clinical lecture thrown in among the huge volume of basic sciences, spicing up the curriculum and making the learning seem more relevant to our careers. Of course, the guest speaker always showed trauma pictures with brains hanging out amid his talking points. I think now it was done on purpose to slowly desensitize us to things we would see in the trauma room.

One story that stands out in my mind was a patient with trigeminal neuralgia. This poor soul presented with chronic, intense pain in the face. Some describe it as a constant and severe cold-freeze similar to what occurs after downing ice cream too quickly. In fact, before modern medicine was developed, a percentage of these patients killed themselves. The surgeon showed the inside of the patient's skull with pictures taken with an endoscopic camera. An artery was wrapped around a nerve and pulsating with each heartbeat. They carefully removed the artery and secured it away from the delicate nerve, making the patient pain-free after that day. Unfortunately, not all causes of trigeminal neuralgia are so easily identified and fixed.

In order to memorize all of this pathology, I went to class during the day and to the library at night. I stayed late every night, studying as hard as I physically could. The morning after the first exam, I noticed the onset of heart palpitations. They began as a significant thumping in my chest every few minutes. By the end of the day, they had increased to a frightening rate of every few seconds. Yet, being the typical medical student, I stayed at the library studying until 11 PM, proving that we are sometimes the last people to admit there may be a problem with our own health.

While I was walking out to the parking lot to go home that night, I called my fiancée Nicole and described the situation to her. She made me go straight to the ER, which

I probably should have done in the first place. I stayed in the ER until early in the morning without seeing a physician. An exam was scheduled for the following morning and my anxiety about losing sleep began to climb. As a result, I read my own EKG as negative and checked out with plans to follow up in the clinic. Later that week in the clinic, they instructed me to return to the ER if the symptoms returned. Of course, the palpitations started again late one night, and I had to return to the ER. I apologized profusely for walking out on them the previous night, since it had to be the same staff working that night. I suppose this is why they tell us not to be our own physicians in the future. We can't seem to be objective when diagnosing and treating ourselves.

Everything turned out fine, thankfully. Since stress played a major role, I had to learn to deal with the heart palpitations for a few months until they disappeared. I think the reason I was in denial is because I didn't feel stressed mentally. As a new physician, I wanted to be invulnerable and invincible. I wanted to be the resident physician working forty hours straight without so much as a wink of sleep. I believe that everything happens for a reason. I soon cut back enough to give my body a rest and finished neuroscience with honors.

Mechanisms of human disease, or pathology, started after neuroscience and along with pharmacology, comprised the rest of second year. They were challenging courses with the most information to process and memorize so far in my studies. Many who have gone through the system use the analogy of trying to drink from a water hydrant: the flow seems impossible to maintain but somehow we manage. Every day it piles on more and more while we try to explain to our family and significant others why we can't see them more often. While I learned about thousands of diseases that year, one in particular has made an impression on me. Lesch-Nyhan is a metabolic disorder characterized by both mental and physical developmental abnormalities. Unfortunately, that is not all that caregivers have to worry about. Before the age of five, patients begin to self-mutilate, generally beginning with lip and finger chewing but sometimes progressing to other forms of abuse. All of this was fascinating, yet sad, to me. I couldn't understand how a genetic disease with real physical components could cause such a psychiatric disturbance. I can still recall my professor describing how these patients do not enjoy mutilating themselves. In fact, they dread it just as you and I would. They can't stop, however, and often need to be restrained.

Although the metabolic disorders are very difficult to master, we did not spend much time on them. We had to move quickly through every organ system and learn about the hundreds of diseases that affect each one of them. Pathology all the way down to the molecular level, such as microscopic alterations of cell membrane ion channels, had to be memorized.

Loyola has also instituted a course called Patient Centered Medicine to get us away from the books and teach us more relevant topics in medicine. PCM in our first year focused on learning how to take a good medical interview, while second year focused more on the physical exam. They hire standardized patients, or actors, to act like a patient with a specific illness. We would not know much going into the room during our timed clinical exams other than name and age. Afterward, the "patients" would give us feedback on our professionalism and other doctor skills.

This is the time in medical school where we learn how to do the embarrassing exams such as genital, rectal, and breast. Beginning in the fall of second year, we had to watch videos on how to perform each exam on both sexes. We were then split into groups of four, meeting two standardized patients in a room. One "patient" would be the practice subject while the other explained to us what we may have been doing wrong. They would make us start from the beginning and act just as if it were a real patient encounter. Through this procedure, they monitored what we said and did under pressure, alerting us to unintentional embarrassing moments, such as saying phrases that might be misconstrued as sexually offensive. For instance, we were advised not to say, "Ok, now I'm going to feel your breast." Instead, we were to say, "Ok, now I will begin palpating your breast." It was also not okay to say, "Everything feels good" during a vaginal exam. No further explanation needed.

Actually, the breast exam is quite easy. We practiced on plastic models ahead of time, which prepared us a little bit. Most of the learning came from actual breast palpation on these actors. It takes quite a person to volunteer for such an activity. Well, it's not actually volunteering since they get paid quite well, but it is still something. For the breast, you use your finger pads in a vertical motion until the entire breast and underarm are palpated. In actual practice, most of us quickly abandoned this technique for a circular motion, which executes more naturally for lump detection.

The gynecological exam was done in a similar fashion. One female actor walked us through the steps while we practiced on the other one. I heard that these teams of actors go from school to school so they are very experienced. I couldn't feel the cervix on my patient until she told me, "My uterus is off to the left." Yes, she must have done it before. It's not too abnormal for the uterus to be displaced slightly to one side. For the male exams, the rectal (prostate) and male genital exams were performed at the same time on the same guy. One elderly man had four of us do both exams on him, one right after the other. What surprised me the most is how educated these patients were in the technique. We were being very gentle with this man's testicles until he told us we weren't doing it right and needed to palpate harder. I guarantee a real patient would never say this, which, I suppose, is one great reason to use standardized patients. In addition to palpating the testicles for lumps, one must check for hernia by sticking a finger upwards and out, while having the patient cough. If a hernia or bowel is present, traveling into the scrotum via a weak spot in the abdominal wall, it can be easily felt.

One of the most unpleasant exams to perform is also one of the most important ones for the older male: the rectal exam. While I'm sure no one would choose this subject for leisurely reading, I don't want you to miss out on any of the glorious experiences a medical student goes through. To perform the rectal, you first have the guy drop

15

his shorts and bend over the table. After donning gloves (double gloves for the faint at heart) and lubricating your finger, you insert it into the rectum as far as it will go. In this position, the prostate gland should be in the down position, feeling like a small bump with a small crease in the middle. Any hard bumps or pain on palpation could mean cancer or infection. Polyps in the rectal vault can also be felt if close enough. This could mean the difference between life and death.

From what I have told you thus far you must think that PCM is a class only for learning genital exams. In reality, these were a very small part of our training. The vast majority of PCM involved learning how to handle difficult patients, mastering the history and physical, and learning to interpret x-rays and electrocardiograms (ECGs). Most of us bemoaned the extra work while having to put extraordinary hours into our basic science classes. However, we agreed that the concepts taught in PCM were far more important for our careers than the steps of the Krebs cycle. Unfortunately, grades are what get young doctors into the residency of their choice. So nothing will ever change until the first two years become Pass/Fail without the detailed ranking system.

One of the best parts about PCM was actually getting into the hospital. We would sport our white coats and ties and follow a particular attending around for an afternoon. It was a real treat for those of us who had been studying nonstop for months on end. My facilitator was board-certified in internal medicine and pediatrics. He took us along, and we rounded on interesting patients on his service. One particular patient still firmly fixed in my memory was a girl about four years old who had a disorder characterized by ascending paralysis that started in her feet and continued up her body. I remember entering her room, seeing her lying there, her mother and aunt close by. By the time we arrived, she could hardly move her entire body. The leading theory was a reaction to her steroid medications, although a viral illness could have certainly been the cause. The attending took a few minutes to teach each student how to check for reflexes. We had already been taught how to check for them, but here was the chance to check our skills on a patient with pathological responses.

I could only imagine how scared she and her family must have been, yet she was so polite, smiling the entire time. I couldn't help but think that if I were in her position I wouldn't be nearly as happy as she was. I have always heard about patients who stunned doctors with their uncanny ability to withstand stress and illness, but I never thought I would see it from a pre-school girl. As we left the hospital room, we talked to the resident taking care of her. Luckily, she reported that they all felt she would fully recover from her paralysis. One can never be certain, but it was good to hear. I appreciated those clinical experiences thrown in the midst of years one and two. It helped all of us to remember for what and for whom we were actually studying.

Another one of my excursions into the hospital was for a complete interview with a patient. Somehow I got connected with an elderly woman in the hospital for something I now can't even recall. In those days we gullible first and second year medical students would spend over an hour doing a history and physical on a patient, mainly because we couldn't break from a talkative patient. I can't even imagine doing that now. There aren't enough hours in the day to spend that amount of time with each patient. During my questioning, I checked the family members' history, asking about their health and what caused their deaths.

My ultimate goal was deciphering if there were any diseases in the family that could be hereditary. However, while questioning this woman about her children, I discovered that one of her sons had died as a teenager from unknown causes, under mysterious circumstances. This happened over thirty years before, but she soon began crying as she told me all about him. She told me that the pain really never goes away when you lose a child. I left there that day, one of my first trips to the hospital, with a lot of sadness. Here a disease was taking her life, but she was depressed about something that happened many years ago. I pondered if the pain was worse because she herself was getting close to death. Perhaps she simply wanted all of her children at her bedside to say their goodbyes.

I left all of my early trips to the hospital with a lot on my mind because I had never really seen sick patients before, something I remember telling my father on the phone one day after visiting the hospital. When patients are close to death, they become cachectic, a term that means to waste away. Every sinew and bone protrudes, making the skin appear as if it is merely draped upon their body. I quickly learned to deal with the emotion of seeing so much suffering, or so I thought at that time.

By the end of the year, I was spending most of my time in the books. Many times I left Loyola late at night. Since I usually parked on the top floor of one of the garages, I had a pristine view of the Chicago skyline at night. To me, watching the skyline at night is serene, peaceful. It helped keep things in perspective as I would contemplate on where my life was going. Years were slipping by and much of my life had been consumed with studying. What helped the most to get through the difficult times was Nicole. Although it was difficult planning a wedding at the end of second year, Nicole had taken on the brunt of the responsibility and did most of the planning for the wedding herself. This hope for the future made life even more exciting: I was soon going to have someone to come home to every night.

The United States Medical Licensing Exam Step 1 is arguably the most important test of a medical student's career. It is the test that every student gives his or her all to, since residencies use it to select candidates. Do poorly on Step 1 and you might not get into the specialty of your choice. Deciding to take the safe route, I began studying early in the second semester of my second year. Beginning with fifteen minutes per day before my class work, I slowly built up to two hours per day.

After finals I had one month to cram nonstop for the test. I began the month by taking a small practice exam to see where I was. My score was estimated to be around the national average for actual test takers. My studying throughout the semester had paid off; but, instead of causing me to relax, achievement such as this motivated

18

me to work even harder. That must be a personality quirk of mine. During the same month, I also moved, got sick, got injured working out, and made preparations for my wedding. I was a nervous wreck, to say the least. After reviewing material from the entire first two years of medical school in three jam-packed weeks, I took one more practice test to estimate my progress.

I had gained over thirty points on my score, which placed me in the top fifteen percent. I bore down on the last week with hundreds of practice questions. No more reviewing and reading slowly. It was time to cram with questions similar to the exam, only with multi-paragraph explanations. Before I knew it, the monster I had feared so long was over, and, soon after, I had the greatest wedding to the most wonderful wife. Honeymooning in Hawaii made me forget all about my troubles for a short time. We returned home and settled into our new apartment. When I received my test score months later, I had received a 256. Since percentiles were no longer given on test results, I had to inquire from some educated physicians how good the score actually was. It turned out to be around the ninety-fifth percentile among all medical students in the country. It was time for celebration!

While everything seemed to be falling into place, I now had to prepare for what would be one of the most difficult years of my training. The basic science years were officially over and the clinical years were about to begin.

Chapter 3: Third Year: The Core Rotations

The rest of my book will detail the experiences I had while rotating through specific specialties during third and fourth year. The vast majority will focus on the surgical months because that's where my interest is. I did want to touch on some of the most interesting key events from the primary care months.

The order of my third year was the following: six weeks of both psychiatry and family medicine followed by three months of internal medicine; six weeks of both obstetrics/gynecology and pediatrics followed by three months of surgery. Everyone rotates through these same core specialties. Some argue that third year is the most difficult year of medical school while others say second year is harder. I think it just depends on which is more challenging, studying nonstop or working nonstop. Personally, I enjoyed third year because I finally began to feel like a physician-in-training.

The surgical months were the most difficult of medical school, but I actually enjoyed them. You are truly the bottom of the totem pole as an MS3. While the first and second years are hiding out in the library all the time, third year allows you exposure and visibility to the rest of the hospital. Nervously finding your way through the maze of knowledge and hierarchy is an unsettling, vicious cycle. If, by chance, you begin to feel comfortable after a month or two on a rotation, this is brought to an abrupt end as you start another rotation and start from scratch. Still, I hope this information doesn't scare away any readers who are pre-med. If you are ambitious enough to get into medical school, you can certainly hack it. The challenge of getting accustomed to new physicians and patients with different expectations is only one more hurdle you have to jump on your way to attaining your medical degree.

Before we were allowed to set foot inside the hospital, we had to be taught the basic procedures we might be performing. Among these procedures was inserting an IV for access to a vein. We gathered in the basement anatomy lab that was eerily vacant of the dead bodies we were used to seeing. It seems strange to describe the absence of dead bodies as eerie, but that's medical school for you. After breaking up into small groups, we practiced putting the IV's into each other. A few students couldn't stomach being poked with a needle so some of us were poked multiple times. It's a little daunting to think that physicians out there can be afraid of needles, reminding me what I've heard time and time again... that doctors often make the worst patients. Anyway, we were taught the steps of the procedure and then the fun began. I had to wait awhile for my turn so I got to watch the situation unfold as a spectator.

I am certain that if the public had seen us that day, their confidence in us as future doctors would have been shaken. Puddles of blood collected underneath a number of tables as certain steps were missed or neglected. Imagine waiting for your turn at such an event. Nevertheless, we all had fun with it; and, luckily for me, my partner seemed to be quite good at it. No pints of blood were lost from me that day. When it was my turn to practice, I placed the tourniquet on my colleague's arm and felt for the best vein possible. Finding this perfect vein in some individuals can be quite difficult. Still, I quickly found my target and punctured the skin with my needle. To my disbelief, I saw no blood in the needle. I knew I had to begin digging around to find the elusive vein.

First, I pulled back and angled to the right before plunging the needle deeper into his flesh. When this didn't work, I tried the other direction. Fortunately, after only a few tries, I found the vein and punctured it with my needle, my partner breathing a sigh of relief at this point as well. This was a small but significant victory for me, the first of many procedures that I would be called upon to do in my medical training. No matter how small or insignificant the task at hand is in medical school, a sense of accomplishment accompanies it.

Towards the end of my third year we had a similar workshop involving a number of different procedures.

These included placing a Foley catheter in the bladder to drain urine and a catheter through the nose to drain the stomach, as well as drawing an arterial blood gas. Thankfully, these were practiced on plastic models this time instead of each other. The only catch is that we were timed at each station with a physician watching and grading our every move. This practice session was so successful that Loyola considered adding it to the beginning of third year. Most of us had already logged numerous procedures by the end of third year and felt it would be more helpful as an introductory course similar to the IV session.

As I reflect on my experiences over the first two years, I realize how far I really came. If asked if I would ever want to repeat any year of medical school, I would reply a quick and emphatic "No!" Although I enjoyed myself, overall it was one of the biggest challenges of my life. Yet, while the hours were long and the grading was difficult, I still have no regrets. I met a lot of interesting people who made a lasting impact on my life and career. I hope you enjoy the stories that follow in the remaining chapters of this book. My sincere desire is that they affect you as much as they have me and that the change is a positive one.

Chapter 4: Psychiatry

With the basic science years behind me, it was time to transition into the clinical years. I performed my six-week rotation in psychiatry in the suburbs of Chicago at a small behavioral health center, an intermediate center where patients were transitioned through the facility on a short-term basis. Really sick patients who are a danger to society are kept under lock and key at long-term care facilities. The students who rotated at these facilities informed me that they had to wear a belt with an alarm when they entered patient-care areas. Because of isolated areas in the facility, the alarms were used in case of an attack. In such a case, safety procedures required them to activate the device and then fall to the floor, covering their ears. Security with ear protective devices would then rush into the area and subdue the combative patient.

Although my facility wasn't as intense as this, precautions still needed to be taken. On the first day I was given a key chain to get through all of the locked doors into the areas where patients resided. I primarily worked with an addiction specialist and learned about the difficulties of weaning people off drugs and alcohol. Occasionally, when I was assigned a psychotic patient, I had to overcome my own personal fears in order to see and learn from a suffering patient. When I arrived the first morning, I paged the attending to let him know I had arrived. He told the secretary to send me to the second floor, as they were about to begin electrical shock therapy. I nervously made my way through the locked doors and, after asking directions a couple of times, found my destination. The attending and resident had already sedated a patient and were about to begin the therapy.

Electrical shock therapy is probably the most controversial topic in the field of psychiatry. It has been stigmatized by such dramas as *One Flew over the Cuckoo's Nest* and *A Beautiful Mind.* The depiction of beloved

23

characters convulsing in true torture while being held down by half a dozen people doesn't help the public's view of such treatment. Undoubtedly, everyone who has seen Hollywood's depiction is afraid to consent when offered shock therapy.

The truth of the matter is that shock therapy is very effective for certain forms of depression and catatonia. Sometimes clinical depression can become so severe that patients have difficulty moving or getting out of bed. This is the type of pathology that responds best. Despite what Hollywood depicts, psychosis is not generally treated via this method, although it is not an unfamiliar treatment.

When the patient was completely sedated and secured with restraints, probes were placed on each side of his head and an electrical impulse was given to him. His muscles contracted and he convulsed slightly, but it was markedly diminished due to the muscle relaxants given prior to the procedure. The electricity was applied for only a few seconds, yet the brain seized for about half a minute. During this time a machine hooked up to his brain printed out brain waves for the psychiatrist to interpret. I learned that another way to know when the seizing stopped is to watch the feet for cessation of twitching.

In less than a couple of minutes the seizure was over and the anesthesiologist began the process of waking the patient and transporting him to the recovery room. Within seconds, the door opened and another patient was wheeled in for shock therapy. This process went on all morning as I watched patient after patient shocked into a seizure. I found the whole procedure to be nothing like that seen on television and much more humane.

The statistics speak for themselves. Shock therapy is drastically more effective than medications for severe depression. Sadly, most facilities don't use it anymore simply because of the stigma associated with it. I think the medical community needs to step up and do what is right for our patients. A good doctor can explain the risks and benefits to patients and usually guide them down the proper path. I will admit that there are some side effects; short-term memory loss and confusion are many times evident immediately after therapy, but the symptoms usually fade within a few weeks. Another downside is that multiple sessions over a set of weeks may be necessary before progress is seen. This can mean more than ten sessions.

In my first week I saw a patient so catatonic and unresponsive that he could hardly speak. After only one therapy, he could carry on a conversation. In fact, he was shaving when we walked into the room. While he was still a bit confused, his state of mind was better than before.

I was fortunate to be able to witness the shock therapy as an introduction to my psychiatry rotation. Many of my classmates didn't even get to see the procedure because they were rotating at institutions that didn't use it.

After a great start, I had no idea that many more interesting experiences would occur before the rotation was over. I was nearly assaulted once. One young man, belligerent and angry, was cursing the nurses because they wouldn't give him his personal possessions. As he tried to knock a chart over onto the nurse, I grabbed it from him and then naively continued my work. Not many seconds later I realized that he was standing only inches behind me, breathing down my neck and cursing in an attempt to antagonize me. As calmly as possible, I walked around the desk to sit with everyone else, trying to ignore him. This indifference only fueled the flames. He began cursing all the louder and had to be taken into another room by his counselor. On the way by, he knocked a cup over at me. By this time my heart was racing a bit, but I later joked that I could have taken him. He was much shorter than I was, so part of his delirium must have been an exaggerated sense of strength.

During one of my first interviews, I talked with a woman in her late 40's who was accompanied by her husband. As I neared the completion of my meticulous interview, I had nothing more to go on than vague symptoms of depression. As I was leaving, the husband interjected to tell his side of the story, describing her auditory and visual hallucinations. She had taken a mental nosedive, falling headlong into a psychotic break. A strange "man" had been telling her to do things that didn't make sense, such as giving rides to random strangers.

That morning, she had revealed to her husband that she was going to die. With this news, I glanced at her to see a confused look on her face. While she claimed that she had no recollection of ever saying such a thing, the husband stared at the floor, shaking his head in disbelief. This man was overwhelmed by the idea that his wife, this woman he loved, was slipping into a perilous mental state. I quickly summoned the attending psychiatrist and we worked out a regimen of anti-psychotic drugs and counseling therapy. Sadly, I never saw them again after that day. Part of me wishes I could have followed up on all of the patients I saw in my years of training to find out what happened to them.

Between patients, we were required to attend group sessions to see what caseworkers and counselors do on a day-to-day basis. Imagine walking into a small room and sitting in a circle with a group of substance users wearing a pristine white coat. I found it embarrassing at first, but the people there were very friendly and made me feel comfortable. Now that I reflect on it, I am sure they were just as ill-at-ease. Group therapy was the opportunity for patients to have time away from the physician to relax and open up. My being there probably represented a physician status. I hope my presence didn't inhibit their progress in any way.

Another counselor I shadowed was a specialist in adolescent psychology, which consisted mainly of eating disorders. The room was filled to capacity with young girls and one boy who had an array of illnesses such as anorexia, bulimia, and depression. The one fact I came away with that day is how deadly eating disorders are. Our society too often shrugs it off as an adolescent phase of fitting in and losing weight, but it is no such thing. Anorexia carries a ten-percent mortality rate, astronomical in medical terms. We need to face this dilemma as a society and confront the distorted way we view body image.

Anxious to get back to one-on-one patient interaction, I decided that one day in the different small groups was enough for me. Later that week the attending told me to interview a new patient in the high security ward. As I walked up to greet him there at the end of the hallway, he seemed like a pleasant, middle-aged man with a genuine smile. After warming him up briefly with some small talk, I began to engage him as to why he was hospitalized there. He opened up to me immediately about the events that led to his arrest and subsequent hospitalization. A few months earlier it came to his attention that a particular truck driver was a convicted pedophile. At first he was not alarmed by this information; however, when he realized that one of his stops was in the immediate vicinity of a child daycare center, he became very concerned. Since a family member ran the trucking service that employed this man, he immediately brought him up to speed on the situation, imploring his relative to terminate his employment before something bad happened. He was distressed when his relative continued to ignore his pleas to take action.

After months of being ignored, his anxiety level grew to the point that he was contacting the police with letters and phone calls, to no avail. No one but him seemed to care about the danger this pedophile posed to those innocent, young children. In fact, his family became angrier with him about his persistent pleas, finally driving him to a point of desperation. He mailed an angry letter to his family, reminding them of the gun he had and that things were going to get ugly if they didn't listen to him. The patient was promptly arrested and placed temporarily in the psychiatric hospital for a psychiatrist's evaluation.

Let's now take a step back. I presented the story to you as the patient told it to me. I learned very quickly in psychiatry that psychotic patients can present themselves as rational people. The difficulty lies in deciphering fact from fiction. As he told me this story, I was nearly convinced of his point of view. There may have been no pedophile at all, but I had no way of knowing from my fifteen minute conversation with him. The person referred to by the patient could have been a completely normal person with no criminal background or not even exist at all. In the end, he was clearly psychotic, and treatment was initiated for his sickness.

Psychosis is not limited to older individuals. Another patient I saw on the same ward was a young man in his twenties. He was well-educated in biology and even in

27

psychology. Consequently, he knew as much as I did about his diagnosis of bipolar syndrome. In conjunction with a psychiatrist, his family had admitted him against his will just a week prior. This did not go over very well with him, since he was as convinced of his sanity as you and I would be about our own. To get him off defense, I began asking him about his personal life. He went on to tell me about his studies at a major university and how he left it to pursue a career as a musical agent. He was representing an up-and-coming rapper in no time at all. The money began to pour in, and he had to fly all across the country to make business deals. He called his family during one of these "business trips" to inform them he would be visiting in a few days. They seized this opportunity to set up an appointment with a psychiatrist. It was tricky getting him to the appointment, but they carefully managed.

When they realized they were not getting through to him, the parents and psychiatrist left the room. Only the physician returned with the help of two assistants. They physically forced him into the facility as he begged and pleaded with them to believe his side of the story. While he was telling me all of this, I couldn't help but look at this young guy with pity. He reminded me of one of my good friends, which made the scenario all the more surreal. Once again I was confronted with a very sick patient who could have convinced me of his side of the story up until the very end of the conversation. I left there convinced that the field of psychiatry is not as simple as I had envisioned it would be.

Bipolar syndrome is the new name replacing manic-depressive disorder. Patients can seem totally normal for long periods of time before going into highs that can last for days or even weeks. Inflated ego (like being an important music agent), impressive spending sprees (like traveling across the country), and high-rolling gambling are just a few of the symptoms patients can manifest. The drop-off from the high can be intense. Depression following the highs leads to an astonishing rate of suicide and substance use among these patients. This fact underscores the need for careful management of anyone with this diagnosis. Lithium has long been the treatment of choice.

28

No one really understands why this element works so well but none can argue against its effectiveness. It likely enters the nerves similar to the sodium ion and works in that regard. It is noted, however, to have many side effects. Fortunately, with the recent boom in the pharmaceutical industry brought about by capitalism, new and better agents are being produced. Hopefully, progress will continue and these patients can lead normal lives.

One misconception I had about third year was that I would be functioning similarly to a resident and that lectures would finally be over. Because psychiatry was very heavy on lectures, I had to drive back to Loyola for half-day lectures two-to-three times per week. Luckily, the rest of the year wasn't as bad. The drive from my institution to Loyola was about forty-five minutes. This really cut into the already short amount of time I had to learn about psychiatry. It wasn't all for nothing though. The lectures supplied us with the difficult psychopharmacology material we needed for the exam.

During my rotation I also had to take three nights of call at Loyola. I remember the first call very well because it was my first time sleeping at the hospital. In-hospital psychiatry is very different from private practice or smaller facilities. Psychiatrists take consultation in-house for a variety of conditions including drug-induced delirium, suicidal ideation, and combative behavior. My first patient ever while on-call was a patient in the thoracic ICU. No one seemed to know who he was or what he was doing there. The emergency department had run out of beds downstairs so they dumped him in the only bed they could find. By this time, he had been given so many sedatives I couldn't even wake him up to ask him questions. I believe most of these medications were given at an outside institution before transfer. At the time, however, I didn't know if the drowsiness was drug-induced or pathological.

I would round on him, talk to the nurses, and then leave to perform other duties that I was responsible for. Later on in the night I would stop by to see if he could be roused. Unfortunately, I left the next day before he ever came out of this state. Consequently, I never even got to talk to my first on-call patient.

I had many other patients to see, though. I talked to two suicidal patients in the ER. One was bipolar and came in because he felt a manic episode coming on and wanted to be protected. I found it very interesting that he could sense the mania and had the good judgment to seek help. The other guy was a homeless man who tried to throw himself in front of traffic. One of the residents and I tried to talk to him but didn't get very far. He was overcome with depression and needed to be hospitalized overnight. Institutionalization would likely follow.

During my last call we were consulted on a pregnant woman who was addicted to heroin. Since she was going through withdrawals, we needed to come up with a drug regimen to prevent her and her baby from getting too sick. Her appearance was extremely rough and haggard. After we talked for a while, she began to spill her story. After finding out she was pregnant, she had decided early on to abort the fetus. Not until she heard the baby's heart beat on Doppler did she change her mind. At that moment she realized she had a beautiful life growing inside of her, and something inside her clicked. She decided to get clean and raise her baby in a better life than what she had known. Although I still feared for the baby from a medical standpoint, I was happy that she had begun the process of changing her life for the better.

My very last patient at the suburban hospital was a memorable one as well. He was a young guy no more than twenty years old, suffering from depression and substance abuse. During the interview, I asked him about the scrapes and cuts all over his arms and face. He freely explained how he had sat out on his grass in his front lawn and had begun cutting himself with a pocketknife. He also had put his cigarettes out in the wounds. Not only did he cut himself, but he took the tip of the blade and tore out little chunks. It was punishment for whatever crime plagued his troubled mind. The phenomenon of cutting has grown in rapid popularity in today's youth. They describe it more as a way to feel something because they are so numb with depression. Apparently, pain is preferable because they at least feel something and know they are alive. I can't explain it any better than this because I don't understand it myself. Apparently, it is very common in the adolescent girls with eating disorders. An entire book could be written on this subject alone. So, my rotation in psychiatry ended on a disturbing note, to say the least. I turned in my keys and began preparations for my next rotation. Having my first rotation of third year over and done with was pretty exciting. I learned a great deal about psychiatric illness and the medicines used to treat them. The field is far from perfect, though, and a lot more needs to be learned about the mind and its relationship to the body. Hopefully, we will see much more advancement in the years to come.

Chapter 5: Family Medicine

At first I thought I would be bored with my rotation in Family Medicine, but the variety of patients and pathology allowed for much enjoyable interaction with residents in ER, Dermatology, Gynecology, and Pediatric clinics. I actually experienced more outpatient procedures here than in any other rotation during third year. When there were minor skin lesions, such as warts, I burned them off with liquid nitrogen or acid. I also performed gynecological examinations, including biopsies of cervical lesions.

I performed the cervical biopsy on a patient much younger than I. After inserting the vaginal speculum, I placed a camera in front of the vagina to project the view onto a monitor, swabbing peroxide on the cervix to lighten up lesions that had been picked up on her previous Pap smear. Peroxide dehydrates the mucosa causing squamous cell lesions to appear white in color, a lesson the attending physician emphasized for accurate tissue biopsy. She handed me an instrument with a sharp clamp at the end. I was to push in, clamp the handle, and withdraw the sample for pathological review. For the first time, I was able to perform a significant procedure, actually simulating what I had learned from lecture and textbook. I was adamant with myself about one thing: I was not going to fail.

My zealous ambition caused me to push a little too hard. A substantial piece of cervix was inadvertently offended, causing her uterus to go into a brief spasm similar to a severe menstrual cramp. The discomfort lasted only a few seconds, and the procedure was over, completing my work schedule for that day. Later, I saw the pouring-down rain streaking the glass as I approached the corridor doors to go home. Before I could exit, I saw the same young girl waiting by the doors, and I felt a wash of awkward dilemma. I chose to face the pouring rain.

While a large percentage of patients had chronic complaints, such as high blood pressure and diabetes, occasionally a patient would come in with a different complaint.

When a young, college-aged female came in to simply get a physical, I was admittedly mystified. I talked with her a little bit about her health and examined her briefly. On the abdominal exam, I noted some tenderness upon palpation of her lower abdomen. As a curious third year medical student, I probably spent a little too much time poking around on my new find. I subtly mentioned my finding during my presentation to the resident but didn't dwell on it. The resident and I went over the topics common to a young female during our encounter. When time for the breast exam arrived, the resident wanted to teach her how to do it herself; and, after some awkward moments, I was sent out of the room. Considering the fact that a few decades ago most physicians were male, I find this common occurrence a bit ironic and a lot detrimental, as it is without a doubt hurting our training. Nevertheless, I replied that I would get the proper equipment to check her hearing while I was outside.

I must have returned too quickly because, when I entered the room, they were engaged in conversation about abortion. At first, I didn't understand how that subject had come up, but I quickly connected it to her abdominal pain. She had just had an abortion but was too ashamed to tell me to stop palpating around on her belly. I think "getting a check-up" was her way of seeing if she was recovering well, and I wondered if the resident had been male if she would have brought it up at all. Checking her ears now seemed stupid, but I did it anyway, mainly because nothing else was left for me to do. The resident gave her the "We're-always-here-if-you-need-to-talk-to-someone" bit, but it did nothing for her. I could see it in her eyes: she was suffering. I suppose you can eventually get over the initial pain, but you can never truly forget it.

She was the last patient we saw that morning. That afternoon was dermatology clinic, and an attending came to teach us special disease cases of the skin. It was a sight to behold.

With residents and medical students there, each patient had to describe his or her problem before more than a dozen people. One middle-aged woman complained of severe itching, so severe, in fact, that she said that she could "understand how people could kill themselves if they couldn't stop this itching." We learned from the dermatologist that such extreme itching without corresponding physical signs usually points to one thing: scabies, a highly-contagious condition. We scraped her skin onto a slide and put it under the microscope. Although the specimen was difficult to see, we saw definite critters on the slide, all of us nearly gagging at the sight and thought of it. Although the room was crowded with over a dozen people, fortunately, none of us contracted the bug, as far as I know.

One of the patients that day had a peculiar rash on his neck that mystified even the dermatologist, a specialist of twenty years. I could only imagine the apprehension the patient could be feeling at this point. So, when physicians don't know exactly what to do, we biopsy. The resident retrieved a small cylinder-like device, the end of which was razor sharp. After numbing the area with local, he placed the cylinder over the rash and pushed down while twisting it back and forth, cutting an "O" into the patient's skin. He used scissors to cut the fascia underneath it and placed the sample in a container to be sent to pathology. The process seemed fairly straightforward to me. I was hoping that if another biopsy came up, they would let me do it. It didn't happen.

The family physician sees common complaints that are musculoskeletal in origin. Arthritis is usually the culprit. Although we can't cure run-of-the-mill osteoarthritis yet, we can ameliorate it with injections into the joint for lubrication and anti-inflammatory effect. The residents must have liked doing these procedures because I saw all kinds of shoulders, knees, and even feet being manipulated. Once again the poor third year was left out of the action. Watching had to suffice for now. This was not the only rotation where this was the case. A physician once told me that he would "teach" me how to inject a knee if I showed up early the following morning. My only reward for arriving early turned out to be watching him do everything. What a letdown that was, a feeling familiar to every medical student.

One should not be concerned by the medical students' eagerness to perform painful procedures. Actually, we're a bit apprehensive about the fact that, in a few years, we will be practicing physicians. This epiphany causes constant reflection on where we are in our training and if we have enough experience. If we're not careful, we could go through medical school with minimal or no hands-on experience. This is unacceptable even for those students who will not enter a surgical specialty.

The gynecology clinic was at an underserved Hispanic clinic where most patients were females, 18-25 years of age, wanting birth control. In order to get the prescription, they needed a yearly gynecological and breast exam. I learned a lot of skills that day, quite an advantage for me as a male medical student since more women are now requesting female physicians. Back-to-back exams for an entire afternoon allowed me to leave there feeling confident in my gynecological skills before the ob/gyn rotation even started. Rather than performing a certain procedure sporadically, I was able to refine and correct my mistakes in the span of a few hours. I would go into the room and interview the patients to get the basic information. One of the female residents or attendings would then come in and chaperone me as I performed the pelvic and breast exam. When appropriate, the attending would double-check my work but never identified me as only a medical student.

The female exam is actually quite simple. The breast exam must include the axilla, or underarm, since most breast cancers drain through this lymphatic system.

For the pelvic exam, I inserted the lubricated speculum into the vaginal canal. Squeezing the handle of the speculum opened the canal, thus giving a good view of the cervix. Since this was a free clinic with limited funds, we had to shine a lamp into the canal to aid in visualization. Later on in the year when I rotated at Loyola, the speculums had built-in lights that illuminated the canal, an upgrade not unlike going from a Honda to a Benz.

The Pap smear is a test used to detect cervical cancer or pre-cancerous lesions. Since this type of cancer is caused by a sexually transmitted disease, HPV (Human Papillomavirus), we test for it in women as young as eighteen or whenever the patient is sexually active. For this test I inserted a brush with a pointed tip into the small hole in the cervix that leads to the uterus. After twirling it a few times to gather cells, I removed it along with the speculum. A quick bimanual exam would follow with a two-finger insertion into the vagina to palpate for masses or tenderness. Pain in girls this young would signify gonorrhea or chlamydia. A mass would likely represent a cyst or tumor.

I did quite well for the vast majority of patients I encountered that day. Admittedly, they were mostly young, thin women, the kind of patient on which the pelvic exam is easy to perform. Only one patient got the best of me that day, the one weighing nearly 400 pounds. When the attending asked me to do the speculum exam, I nervously considered the difficulty of the case and believed that she should do it. That was not what she had in mind. I believe she wanted me to have one tough case so I would have to troubleshoot my way through it. When the patient was in the Lithotomy position, I tried to insert the speculum. I found myself having difficulty even finding the vagina due to the large pannus, or abdominal fat rolls.

After trying for a few minutes, I became embarrassed for the girl so I blindly slid the speculum in, hoping to find the right spot. I tried a couple of times before giving up and allowing the attending do it, something that no medical student ever wants to do. Giving up is abhorrent to us, probably one of the personality traits that got us into medical school in the first place. Showing off her expertise, the attending was successful on her first try. I'm sure she has performed thousands of them so I had nothing to be ashamed of. We quickly performed the breast exam and sent her on her way.

At the same facility we also had a pediatric clinic where my bewilderment in baby and toddler examination is nothing less than comical. First of all, I had no idea what I was doing since no one ever taught me how to talk to or examine a child. Furthermore, I don't remember any lectures on how to talk to their mothers, an incident exacerbated by the need for a translator to understand half of them. The first mother must have had her faith shaken in the medical community after talking to me. It got better, though; it always does.

One particular woman brought in her young son, an eight- or nine-year-old who had suffered with constipation issues ever since he was three. What finally brought her to the doctor's office was the fact that he was being teased at school for smelling like feces. An exam revealed that his rectum was full of stool, which consequently soiled his underwear. Her explanation of the etiology was unsatisfactory. After questioning her in greater detail, I learned that his constipation problems began when his younger sibling was born. Toddlers will often revert to a more immature psychological level when they feel jealous of a younger sibling. The situation never went away on its own as the parents hoped it would. I can only assume the delay in coming to the physician was lack of insurance and possibly legal status. He was placed on a strict regimen of bowel softeners and toilet training. He would have to sit on the toilet for an hour after meals, if needed, to retrain his bowels to work properly. I don't know if the mother followed our advice or not. For the child's sake, I sure hope so.

As the residents and medical students each saw a patient alone and then in concert with the attending, I usually saw only a third of the patients. However, when something interesting came up, all of us would cram into the tiny room to be taught by the specialist, an event usually followed by ten-to-fifteen minutes of huddling around the textbooks reading anything pertinent aloud. One of those episodes presented itself as a very exciting one for me personally, as I was able to make an important discovery through observation.

Gathered in a room where the patient was a one-year-old girl, we were listening intently to the doctor. During the lecture, I looked down to see the child's hair pulsating over the fontanel, the soft spot, an opening between the plates of the skull in young children. I alerted the specialist to my observation, who quickly listened with his stethoscope over the pulsation. After a few seconds, he announced that she had a bruit, turbulence in blood flow in the venous system around the brain. Everyone gathered around to listen to the new discovery. I think I was even high-fived a couple of times. Moments like that in our medical training keep the adventure of uncharted territory exciting, each student hoping to discover something new. It turned out to be nothing serious and not even that rare. I did, however, have my few minutes of glory.

My final clinic rotation was actually no clinic at all, as I served two afternoons in the emergency department. During my first shift, a large burly man came in with rectal bleeding. Apparently upon moving his bowels that morning, he filled his entire toilet with blood. The episode was described as completely painless. I did my history and physical and waited for the attending to present the case to him. Some time had passed as the doctor was seeing another patient at the same time. When we finally went to see the patient together, he told us he just had another bloody bowel movement and saved it for us. Most ER physicians have seen this scenario a million times over and would politely refuse such a disgusting show. However, for my "benefit" we went to the bathroom to make our observations. The toilet was filled with red-black blood clots and the foulest smell imaginable. A nearby technician proclaimed, "Once you smell *that* you will never forget it." And I never have.

Time not spent at the free clinic or the residency center was spent with a private practitioner in the community. My mentor was an osteopathic-trained family practitioner or DO. The DOs complete medical training similar to allopathic MDs, except for a few minor differences, one of which is the concept of manipulation. Manipulation uses the chiropractor's philosophy of physical force to align misplaced joints and discs. The first time I witnessed him in action, I nearly toppled over with disbelief. While the procedure looked painful and frightening, the patients swear by its effectiveness.

Depending on the patient's complaint, the doctor began his procedure by positioning the patient on the table. Keep in mind that these are patients with severe orthopedic complaints. Then, using his full body weight, he snapped, pulled, and jerked their joints into place, a remarkable feat that would cause split-second shouts of discomfort. Shortly thereafter, they left the building with a smile. I'm still not sure I would let him do it to me, but if it works for some, more power to him. Still, snapping someone's neck is no small matter, an art form not learned overnight. It can even cause a debilitating stroke in a small number of patients. The osteopaths spend a significant portion of their time learning their craft. For those not going into primary care, they usually abandon the practice of manipulation shortly after medical school. Regular performance is required in order to maintain the skills.

Even though I didn't perform any manipulation, he let me do other small procedures. My favorite was using liquid nitrogen to burn off warts. One particular case was especially amusing to me, though I have no idea why. One of the patients seemed nervous about allowing me to practice on him. After being asked about his hesitation, he told me that years earlier he had allowed a medical student to do the same procedure; supposedly, the student ended up butchering his hand. How anyone can mess up such a simple task is beyond me. Fortunately, he got over his fear and allowed me to proceed. I never liked to leave a room without fulfilling whatever the physician instructed me to do, my fault or not.

That physician also let me pack a groin wound. This is not the most glamorous job in the world, I can assure you. The guy had an abscess in his groin that wouldn't heal, but he also had poor hygiene. These two factors combined synergistically to produce the most potent odor I had ever smelled, including the aforementioned toilet sample. The first task was to remove the packing placed at the last visit, a near twelve inches of string extracted from a small hole in his skin, it seemed. Next, I cleaned the wound by inserting a Q-Tip dipped in peroxide, moving it in all directions because fistula, or tracts, had developed. In certain areas, I was able to penetrate one to two inches deep. Red bubbles poured out of the wound as the peroxide reacted with the environment. Then I had to redress the wound. I cut gauze into small strips about half a centimeter in width. Using the back end of the Q-Tip, I slowly worked the small strips of gauze into the wound, hoping that the deep wound would slowly heal from the inside out. Keeping it sterile with peroxide would give the body enough time to do just that.

Overall, I enjoyed the family medicine rotation very much. Our country has a definite need for generalists like family doctors. Underserved areas need physicians that can handle multiple problems crossing over multiple specialties. America, however, is moving the way of the specialist, especially with the explosion of science and technology, preventing those in primary care from keeping up with the subtleties of each specialty. My interests at the time were emergency medicine or critical care. I knew I wanted a procedure-oriented field, but I had no clue it would take me as far as a surgical subspecialty. Many surprises were waiting for me over the next few months that would forever change my life. My anticipation mounted at the end of family medicine.My rotation in internal medicine was about to begin. It was time to take care of really sick patients in the hospital. I was finally going to get some real action.

Chapter 6: Internal Medicine

Most internal medicine physicians work in clinics all day similarly to a family practitioner. The training, however, consists mostly of adult inpatient management. I spent two of my three months in the hospital taking care of extremely ill patients. On my first day at a local community hospital, I thought I was in for a world of change. The medicine team took rapid response calls any time emergencies occurred in the hospital. I had barely gotten my feet wet when a code was called. I ran to the room that was announced over the loud speakers and watched an elderly woman die. She was DNR, do not resuscitate, so all we did was give medications to revive her. No violent chest compressions and ventilators were administered for her. Her time had come and she went peacefully.

What many people don't realize is how nasty reviving someone can really be. The chest compressions often break the ribs in multiple places. I've heard people describe it as doing compressions on a bag of potato chips when the victim is an elderly person. Intubating, or passing a breathing tube down one's throat, can be an equally miserable experience. Patients will often awake in the intensive care unit and be unable to breathe or speak on their own. Some patients who have been intubated in the past will allow for chest compressions in the event of a code, but not intubation. Add to this the fact that we are hardly ever successful in resuscitative effort.

Only a couple of hours later, we responded to another rapid response announcement. This time, we were presented a sight not too dissimilar from a horror movie. The man on the bed was covered from head to toe with blood, his sheets saturated and the floor splattered. Taking charge and barking orders to the nurses, the resident immediately took off her white coat and asked for a nasogastric "NG" tube. She lubricated the tubing and began sliding it down his nose to the stomach, hooking it to the suction device onto the wall. Blood immediately began collecting in the suction box, confirming the diagnosis of an upper gastrointestinal bleed. The patient was transferred to the ICU for closer monitoring.

During this performance, I stood in the corner of the room with a deer-in-the-headlights look, watching the scene before me unfold. After things had calmed down, I asked some questions, first wanting to know how she assessed the situation so quickly and how she knew which procedure to perform. Apparently, she was already familiar with the patient and had seen him vomit blood before. Still mesmerized by her abilities, I realized that I had a very long way to go in my training.

Everything that followed that first day was relatively anti-climactic. The pace slowed to the usual chronic, detailed management of patients in the hospital. Despite all this, I enjoyed the rotation a lot and learned a great deal. We met every day around noon for grand rounds with one resident presenting an interesting patient he or she had cared for the previous week-- a great way to learn since it was about a real patient interaction. Although the tedious management of dozens of medications was not for me, I applaud medicine doctors for their work. During this month, I had my first inkling that I was more of a surgeon at heart.

Even though the first day was packed with the most adrenaline, it was not the only time I was on the rapid response team. My second week we were called to the obstetrics floor for an emergency where a young woman who had just delivered a baby was barely responsive. Her husband reported seizure-like activity, but this could not be confirmed. We tried our best to get a coherent response from her to no avail.

Seizures are a feared complication of pregnancy although, generally speaking, the seizures can be kept under control with certain medications. This seizure disorder, eclampsia, is associated with other pathological anomalies such as elevated blood pressure. Although the best treatment is to deliver the "foreign body," the baby itself, this is not always possible if the baby is too premature to survive delivery. In this case, the baby had actually been delivered, which is not how I expected to see my first eclamptic patient. As I observed this young woman, I felt compassion for both her and her husband, able only to imagine the tremendous fear he must have been experiencing. Here I stood, a newlywed, somehow seeing my own wife lying on that bed, not really knowing what I would do or feel in the same situation. I knew I could not let my personal feelings interfere, so I quickly composed myself and tried to learn as much as I could from the medicine residents and the patient's obstetrician. The doctors' delay in making a decision was a direct result of their not being certain whether she had really had a seizure, since all they had to go on was the husband's word, and he didn't even speak English. At that point, she lapsed into a seizure, quickly resolving the point in question. Happily, the young mother recovered fully and was reunited with her baby.

Later that week, in one of our daily case presentations, we saw a patient with metastatic lung cancer, the cancer having spread so extensively that the lymph nodes in her neck stuck out like ball bearings. The residents gave me her room number and told me to go palpate her lymph nodes. On the way to her room, I tried to think of a diplomatic way to explain to her why someone she had never seen before was feeling her neck. I didn't want her to feel as if she were a showcase with such atrocious cancer that people were coming from all over the hospital to see her.

I introduced myself as a Loyola medical student and asked how she felt. I asked if I could examine her. She agreed, so I first auscultated her heart and lungs to hide my primary interest in her cancerous lymph nodes. Then I felt her neck, my first time palpating cancer in a real patient. All medical students are taught the different chains of lymph nodes in the body. I kept that in mind as I directed my hands, feeling hard nodules each an inch in diameter up and down her neck. After I reported my findings to the residents, they told me that she had only days to live but was in complete denial. In fact, she would not even discuss the matter with the numerous people who tried to broach the subject about becoming DNR. When someone is terminally ill with no cure in sight, putting all affairs in order can allow that person to die in peace.

Another poignant case I saw involved a different form of cancer. We were called for a consult in the ER for an elderly patient complaining of leg pain after a fall. Entering the room, I immediately noticed the remarkable yellow color of her skin. This development shifted our attention from her complaint of a bum leg to the issue she had obviously avoided for months. The patient stated that she had suffered clay-colored stools for some time. After a thorough assessment, I ascertained that she had no abdominal pain.

After discussing the patient with the residents and the attending, they told me something I have not forgotten to this day: painless jaundice is never a good sign. They guessed that she had either pancreatic or bile duct cancer. Either way, it was a death sentence at an advanced stage, as in her case. At that moment, I recalled her reaction when I had inquired into her family history. She noticeably winced when I asked if she had cancer in the family, probably having known the truth all along. It was later proven to be bile duct cancer. We consulted the GI specialists about stenting the bile ducts open to relieve the jaundice and itching that accompanies it. Early the next morning my resident and I saw the GI fellow and went over to ask him about her.

We stood at the nurse's station roughly fifteen feet from the patient's door. He must have found the situation amusing and remarked how she looked like Frankenstein. I found myself cringing as I prayed the sound waves were not making their way into her room. To make matters worse, he was that type of person who thought he was funny, repeating his jokes several times when no one laughed. I was disgusted at his lack of compassion and caring for the patients he had supposedly devoted his life to healing. I hoped that I would not change throughout the long years of training and become jaded like so many have before me.

This particular man was an exception among the physicians I encountered during my month there. The others always maintained nothing less than the proper level of professionalism. My resident, who was an Asian female, admitted a terminal cancer patient who must have thought that since he was dying, he was no longer accountable for his behavior. During our interview, he directed one suggestive vulgarity after another toward her. Although she once reminded him that he was married, this didn't seem to faze him a bit. As we were getting ready to leave, my resident asked him if there was anything else she could do for him. Pushing his bed tray away from his chair, he looked down at his crotch. I couldn't believe what I was seeing; in fact, no one in the room missed the implication. At that moment, the resident had reached her tolerance limit and effectively reprimanded him, putting an abrupt stop to his inappropriate behavior. While this was a strange patient encounter, to say the least, I learned that he had unresolved family issues that resulted in this kind of behavior, a testament to what can happen when these pervasive issues remain hidden.

Part of the "family issue" mystery began to unravel the following morning when the patient's wife arrived, wanting to speak with us outside of his room. She informed us that she and her husband had decided on a DNR status, regardless of what his children wanted. Furthermore, she specifically instructed us that they were to have no voice in making decisions. Not surprising to us, we learned that they were newlyweds, with the wife on poor speaking terms with his grown children. The law was on her side: the spouse has the legitimate right over children when the patient becomes unresponsive and cannot speak for himself.

The best case scenario was to get the children on board before the patient got to that state. First, my resident assured the wife that we would honor her husband's wish to be DNR. Of course, we would provide care and treatment up until that time. Second, she convinced the wife that she and her husband should talk to his children so everyone was on the same page before a crisis arose. Most importantly, she talked with the patient in private to make sure that he was not being coerced into signing a DNR. We talked to him together, and it was indeed his wish to die. He told us that she married him only to get his house. "Let her have it!" he exclaimed. I left there a bit disheartened, but there was nothing more that could be done.

My next month at Loyola was more structured with three-to-four hour rounds every morning with the attending physician discussing every patient on the service. Included was a weekly evening clinic with an Internal Medicine specialist, or internist, a man who boasted a long and successful tenure so everyone knew him by name.

My first clinic with him lasted only a few hours, but I will never forget it as long as I live. I was busy seeing a patient when he opened the door and told me to follow him. I excused myself from the patient interview and accompanied him to another room down the hall. On the way there he informed me that he had found a huge lump on the breast exam of one of his patients. I knew immediately that this was not going to be a comfortable situation.

As we entered the room, I saw a middle-aged woman lying on the table with a tissue in her hand. Tears were streaming down her face, her eyes swollen and red. He told her that, as a physician-in-training, I needed to be able to palpate this tumor so I would never miss it. After she agreed, I began to examine her right underarm and breast using the technique I had been taught in one of my previous classes. To my dismay, I could not feel the tumor even when I knew it was there. He instructed me to try again. That's when I felt my first breast lump, rubber-textured and large in terms of cancerous lymph nodes.

We had her sit up, and he began counseling her. Sitting there with tears in her eyes, she tried to absorb all of the information, so distracted, in fact, that she failed to cover herself. For probably the first time in her life, modesty was the last thing on her mind. The doctor explained that the possibility of chemotherapy, radiation, and even death lurked around the corner. I was a little overcome with the situation, the anxiety level continuing to rise steadily. At that moment, while talking to her about the plan, he embraced her and planted a fatherly kiss on her on forehead. I had never seen such passionate care delivered so eloquently at just the right time. The expression on her face changed slightly in that moment from one of dread to one of determination.

We stepped out to discuss the case and allow her to get dressed. My task at hand was to return to the room from which I had abruptly left, acting as if all was right with the world. I resumed the interview with a polite elderly couple who smiled constantly. I smiled back even though it was the last thing I wanted to do. When I stepped out into the hallway, I bumped right into the newly diagnosed breast cancer patient. We both managed an awkward "take care" as she walked by. I never saw her again.

After she left I was still reeling from the situation but had to focus: clinic had to move on. My next patient was a man in for a regular check-up. I heard the physician's directions to "go in and do a rectal on him," leaving me a little flustered, to say the least, since this was my first rectal exam on an actual patient. After asking him all the right questions about his health, the time came when I introduced the delicate subject of checking his prostate. I could feel the temperature of my face in a steady climb. And then, for some odd reason, I told him he had three options: I could do the rectal exam, the physician could do the rectal exam, or I could do the rectal exam followed by the attending to double-check my work. He laughed and said, "No, just you will be fine." I was certainly glad to have the first one over with. It definitely got easier with experience.

On the wards, I was under the instruction of two third year residents in internal medicine. The third year residents were in their final year, making them seem like attendings to me. Still, seniors or not, they had to listen to lecture with me, which I found to be quite ironic, when they seemed to know everything already. One of them had not filled his requirement on a procedure called pericentesis. A Gastroenterology (GI) fellow had a patient with liver disease, so he walked the resident step-by-step through the procedure while we students eagerly watched. When the liver shuts down, fluid begins to back up, the pressure causing fluid to leak into the abdominal cavity. Liters of fluid can be tapped out of the belly of a patient with end-stage liver disease.

Using a maneuver called percussion, the fellow began tapping the patient's abdomen with his fingers. With this old-school technique, he found the perfect place to stick the large needle into the belly without damaging vital organs. The resident took over and pierced the needle into the patient's abdomen very carefully, withdrawing some fluid to be sent to the pathologists for study. If cancer is the problem, they can usually find cancer cells in the fluid. The needle, however, is used only to pierce the skin and fascia. Tubing is then guided over the needle to be left in place for a period of time determined by the rate of fluid being drained.

At this point I was anxious to do my own tap. I had no such luck. I wondered how long I would have to wait before it would be my turn to start performing significant procedures. Here was a third year medical resident still learning how to do the procedures I was ready to begin at that very moment. I quickly learned that the third year of medical school is not about procedures. It's about mastering the history and physical and choosing a specialty.

The first patient I was personally assigned to on the hospital ward was a middle-aged man with upper abdominal pain. He was a tenacious alcoholic who never missed a drink. After checking his serum enzymes, we suspected pancreatitis, as the two most common causes of pancreatitis are gallstones and alcohol. Apparently, he had been hospitalized previously at Loyola for the exact same thing, but the intense pain and near-death experiences were not enough to convince him to stop drinking.

I questioned him a little further about what had initiated the pain. He described drinking a pint of vodka that day while downing a few cheeseburgers from White Castle, a combination I think would give anyone pancreatitis. Of course, he swore adamantly that he was done for good with alcohol. I should have told him that all we had to do was plug his symptoms and lab criteria into a formula, and we could tell him the percent chance that he would leave the hospital in a body bag. Perhaps that would have made an impact in his life, but I doubt it. The attending did make sure to scold him on the drinking. I hope that he stayed clean. He was just a nice guy with some serious problems he needed to resolve. Each additional episode was causing inflammatory damage and would soon be irreversible. Other than supportive care we didn't do much else for him. Rest, intravenous fluids, and nothing-per-mouth are the treatments of choice. The pancreas needs a chance to cool off before making it go back to work digesting food.

The third month of medicine was an outpatient medicine month. During this time I had multiple subspecialty clinics such as GI, cardiology, and rheumatology. These subspecialists completed a three-year internal medicine residency after medical school, followed by a two- to three-year fellowship. The clinics were so specialized I couldn't see patients on my own because I had no idea what was going on. What third year medical student can talk to patients about their pacemakers? The hours were nice, but I was bored by the end of the month. During this month I was also required to do five shifts in the emergency department. Most of emergency medicine is mundane primary care with a hint of urgency to it. In addition, the waiting room is always full of grumbling patients having the worst day of their lives. These are some of the reasons why I decided against a career in ER.

At one point, the gravity of what I was going to see and do while in medical school and residency made a lasting impression. I was typing a note on one of my patients when the door to the trauma room opened, giving me a glimpse of what literally left my jaw hanging. A young man lay on a bed with the entire left side of his chest ripped open. Yet, everyone was standing around him doing nothing, which could only mean that the time of death had already been called. Within seconds the door swung shut and the show was over. I didn't have the nerve to go in to see what had happened to that young man, but the grisly scene definitely had an effect on me.

After those shifts in the ER, my internal medicine rotation was over. I took the exam and headed off for Christmas vacation and a week of rest. I was gearing up for the surgical specialties and some of the longest and most intense hours of medical school. I knew I had to be prepared.

Chapter 7: Obstetrics & Gynecology

I will give one more warning about the graphic nature of the events that I will describe in this book. Some of it may be difficult to read, but I hope you learn from these patients the way I did. My life changed forever in the second half of third year. I hope to give you a glimpse of what goes on in hospitals that you may pass by on a daily basis. After Christmas break, I began my rotation in obstetrics/gynecology, a six-week clerkship with different subspecialties included.

The first two weeks were on gynecological oncology, followed by urogynecology and labor and delivery Gyn-onc is the subspecialty that deals with cancer of the pelvic organs. Since it is highly surgical, I scrubbed in on my first surgeries and got exposure to the operating room where the hours became long and intense. A typical day would look like the following.

Arriving at the hospital at 4:30 AM, I pre-rounded on the patients that were assigned to me, with a quick conversation about what happened overnight, any pain or side effects from medications, etc. Following a quick physical examination, I typed a brief note into the computer about the encounter. At 5:30 AM, we students met with the senior residents who basically repeated our work since we were still in training and no one trusted our physical examinations. However, it went much more quickly because we had already recorded the vital signs and presented the patient before entering the room.

At 6:30 AM, we had a morning report that entailed meeting in the cafeteria to go over questions to learn as much as we could for the test. After this, we met with the attending physician and rounded for a third time with him. Finally, when the hospital work was done, it was time to begin the day, meaning either clinic or scrubbing in the OR. On this service I scrubbed into quite a few hysterectomies for either benign reasons (fibroids, heavy

51

menstrual periods) or malignant reasons (ovarian, uterine cancer). If there was a malignancy, we sampled the lymph nodes throughout the abdominal cavity to check for metastatic lesions.

The first patient assigned to me had metastatic ovarian cancer that had spread throughout her body. She was in her fifties but appeared much older due to the wasting effects of cancer. Having had chemo the week before, this poor woman was admitted to the hospital with terrible side effects. She had developed mucositis, a condition where blisters and ulcers develop in the mouth and throat. Unfortunately, this was the least of her problems. Her immune cells dropped, and I began to fear the worst.

As I left for the weekend, I doubted that she would be alive when I returned. Before I left, I went to see her one last time in the ICU. I didn't stay long as the ICU residents were trying to get an arterial blood gas sample. The following Monday I arrived to check on her, one hour too late: she had already passed away. If I had shown up an hour earlier, I would have been the one to find her. I can still see the image of her face from the last time I saw her. She was my first assigned patient that I lost on the wards. Rest in peace, Mrs. P.

The most memorable patient was one seen in clinic my first week. She presented with slight vaginal bleeding but had severe complaints of diarrhea and nausea, month-long symptoms for which she had not sought treatment. We suspected mental instability when she became hysterical with me after appearing quite normal with the attending. However, soon thereafter a large ovarian mass was found in her that was most likely cancer. We all felt bad because we had labeled her as histrionic. The attending could not believe that she missed the tumor on pelvic exam.

Scrubbing in on her operation the following week, I feared it would be a tense situation. However, the tumor couldn't be palpated on pelvic exam even under anesthesia. The attending felt a little justified and the operation went much smoother. With the stomach relaxed, however, the tumor could be palpated in the abdomen. The surgery was an amazing experience, producing a tumor about the size of my head, and we attributed not finding it on exam due to her being overweight. We staged her with lymph node biopsies and closed her up without complication. She went home two days later but needed chemotherapy to make sure the cancer cells were eradicated. I had a younger student shadowing me that day so I really showed him a good time in the OR.

Overall, gyn-onc was an interesting yet demanding two weeks, some of the days lasting twelve to fourteen hours. I began going to bed as early as 9 PM, before my wife even got home from work. We saw each other only about half an hour each week. To add to the stress of the long hours was learning the unwritten rules of the OR. Most of them involve maintaining sterility in the room and providing an infection-free environment, two components that could mean the difference between life and death for a patient. Surgeons also have a reputation for being very strict. I rotated with the most sought-after surgeons, but, even still, I was reprimanded a few times for something as simple as cutting the sutures too slowly.

The surgical procedure with the most amazing technique was a vaginal hysterectomy. These were performed for benign reasons when a minimally invasive approach was the most desirable. Resecting the uterus by prolapsing it through the vaginal canal and cutting it out was amazing to watch. It saved the patient a painful abdominal incision and extended healing time. Unfortunately, many women have too large a uterus to use this method and consequently need the abdominal incision.

The following two weeks I rotated through urogynecology. It was also a surgical subspecialty dealing with pelvic floor pathology. Correcting urinary incontinence seemed to comprise most of the work. I had to talk all day about incontinence with older women who undoubtedly preferred I not be there. Medicine can sometimes be an uncomfortable relationship with people who look to you for help. To do this you must often invade privacy, inquiring about embarrassing personal issues.

On the other hand, the surgeries were just as interesting as gyn-onc. For one patient, we were placing an electrical probe into her sacral nerves through her buttocks, a complicated treatment option for refractory incontinence. In order for this to work, the patient has to be awake during the procedure to let the physicians know when the voltage is high enough to feel.

The patient we operated on was a chronic pain patient that must have had nerve damage from previous operations. We kept using local anesthetic, but it was never enough. The patient was screaming in pain the entire operation. We would cut. She would scream. We would use more local anesthetic. She would be fine for a few more cuts. Then there would be more screaming. Luckily, we had administered an anesthetic agent to blot out her memory of the entire incident. The attending explained that the procedure is not usually that difficult and unsettling. Aside from my shock at seeing such a scenario, the patient should have a much better quality of life.

As nightmarish as that incident was, I put it behind me and looked forward to seeing more cases. In other words, if that did not scare me away from surgery, nothing would. I knew I was getting closer to finding the right career path for myself.

Later that week, I had the younger student that shadowed me come watch a vaginal hysterectomy. I instructed him to use a regular mask with no eye shield because he would not be scrubbing in the surgery. I had no way of knowing that the resident would accidentally cut the uterine artery, sending a stream of blood streaking across the room. It splattered the resident standing next to him though they were five feet from the table. It wasn't long before I saw him sneaking out to grab one of the face shields. I doubt he will ever go without one again!

While attaining much surgical skill during third year was difficult, I learned the most important thing about myself during the rotation: I wanted to be a surgeon. Once I let the attendings know I was interested in a surgical career, they provided more opportunities for me. The most interesting was allowing me to practice suturing and tying knots on the uterus after removing it from the patient since the organ was going to be discarded anyway. This was beneficial, because there is no better way to practice than on real tissue.

They set up a tray for me with a scalpel, suturing material, and a nice, big uterus. I began by splaying it open with a vertical incision exposing the endometrial cavity. Next, I used pickups to hold the edges of the incision and hooked them with the needle in the other hand. It was very awkward at first but I quickly got better with practice. After doing this procedure a couple of times, they let me close my first fascial plane in an abdominal incision. I am so thankful the attending left the room because it was a sorry sight. Sewing on discarded organs is quite different from sewing on an actual patient, and my lack of expertise showed. In fact, it seemed to amuse the entire OR and anesthesia staff as they huddled around to watch the newly discovered entertainment.

I was on labor and delivery for only a week and a half and scrubbed in on a few C-sections and vaginal deliveries. My hope of delivering a little one myself never materialized. While the C-sections, I must admit, were very bloody procedures, I was amazed to see the cute purple babies pop out of the mommy's belly. I was so flustered the first time, I didn't even know the sex of the baby when Nicole asked me that night. I think I was too busy dodging the liters of amniotic fluid gushing out all over my hands and feet. It's surprisingly warm. Amid all the excitement of seeing a new case or learning about a new disease, I found it refreshing to step back and appreciate the creation of a new human being. There is nothing like the miracle of life.

The last week of OB was by far the most difficult. Not only did I have the stress of studying for the shelf exam weighing me down, but I was also working difficult shifts. On the Sunday preceding the exam, I took call for twenty-four hours without any sleep. When I finally arrived home around 7 AM, I kissed Nicole "good night" and slept for about five hours before heading back in.

I was switching to night float on L&D so I had to adjust to working Monday night, which ended up being a fourteen-hour shift. On Tuesday, I could sleep for only a few hours in the late morning because I had to go in early to work on a presentation for the department chair on Wednesday. The Tuesday night shift was short because they would not allow me to stay overnight in order for me to be well rested for Wednesday's classes and presentations. In doing this, though, I had to try and switch my sleep schedule again, which wasn't completely successful.

To top it off, I had one of the meanest residents imaginable. She gave me impossible tasks and then yelled at me in front of the entire nursing staff when I couldn't complete them. The unfortunate thing was that she was a good teacher when she wanted to be. We developed a love-hate relationship from which I decided to learn instead of fight. Okay, I moaned a little. To this day, I still have never met anyone as mean as she and probably never will again. Let me give you some examples.

On my first morning I showed up on time for morning rounds. When the resident arrived, she immediately asked me the number of patients I had already picked up. No student picks up patients without talking to the on-service residents first. So when I replied that it was my first day, she was clearly annoyed. Before the first night was over, she had educated me on my inadequacies as a third-year medical student, a judgment she made after being acquainted with me for only a few hours. At the end of the first overnight shift, my nerves were on edge from constant attack and belittling.

On the second shift she asked me to prepare a presentation during my down time. After many hours of reading articles and looking up the stages of labor, we sat down to go over what I had learned. My stack of papers was carefully underlined and annotated with the order of my presentation. The first sentence wasn't out of my mouth before she ripped the papers out of my hands and made me do the presentation without them. I can understand wanting a student to learn material better by forcing him or her to present without notes, but this was ridiculous. The subject matter was totally foreign to me, and I had only a short amount of time to prepare for something of that magnitude.

The residents can make or break you as a medical student. The attending physicians rarely give you much face time; so much of the evaluation comes from the residents. I could barely contain the anger and resentment in spite of this. Up until that point, my time at Loyola had been completely positive. The moment I decided to let it all go was in the hallway walking to the ER with my team. I was trailing behind and heard her remark about how she made at least half of the previous class cry. I now pitied her more than anything else. I didn't let her get to me anymore. Instead, I worked my butt off.

On my remaining shifts I didn't so much as sit down. When I wasn't working, I read and researched labor topics, and I made sure she knew it. After she criticized me in front of all of the staff, I thanked her for her advice. I tried as hard as I could to kill her with kindness; my effort rewarded in the end with a terrible grade which I'm sure was her doing. At least I can find the situation amusing as I reflect on it now. In spite of it all, I still had some amazing experiences that week, some uplifting and others depressing.

One of the depressing moments came while I was on night float. Around 3:30 AM, a pregnant patient came to the emergency room bleeding from her vagina. The baby was dead. I had to scrub in on the same type of procedure as an abortion. As the physician and resident prepared in the other room, I helped get the woman onto the operating table. After we loaded her on the bed, I noticed a large blood clot had passed out of her vagina. The surgical technicians scrambled to get a specimen container, not knowing if the fetus had passed. It turned out to only be blood and was disposed of.

After scrubbing, we dilated the patient's cervix and inserted a vacuum tube into the uterus. The resident began suctioning out the baby in pieces as I watched tissue mixed with blood passing through the clear tubing. She stopped one time to point out that some of the tissue was black, meaning the baby had probably been dead for a while. She inserted an instrument into the uterus to scrape out any remaining tissue, grabbing my hand to scrape while she moved my hand in the appropriate angles. "The gritty feeling is the uterus", she explained. "It would feel smooth if fetal tissue and placenta were still inside. So we're done." Feelings of grief and sadness weighed heavily on my mind.

In the last hour of the rotation I had the opportunity to assist in a vaginal delivery. Since it was a difficult delivery, I didn't get to personally catch the baby, but I did enough to be satisfied. The patient was a young teenage girl who was so worn out she wouldn't comply with our directions on how and when to push. As a result, the process took much longer than it should have. After the baby's head was wedged in the vaginal canal for a while, the attending walked in and said very bluntly, "I want it out." He then turned and walked out of the room.

This was the cue to the resident to take more drastic measures since the baby wasn't responding well. We ended up using a vacuum technique to literally suction the baby out of the canal. A plunger-like device was placed on the scalp and pumped until negative pressure was produced. This helped to pull the baby out while the mom pushed, a technique that quickly produced a baby boy. I clamped the umbilical cord and suctioned out the baby's mouth while we let the father cut the cord and handed off the baby. The resident instructed me to pull slowly on the cord until the placenta was delivered. I watched for the signs of imminent placenta delivery: lengthening of cord, gush of blood, and a contracting uterus as palpated in the abdomen of the patient.

After the disgustingly ugly mass of tissue and blood was out, I had to inspect it to make sure no pieces had torn off inside the uterus since any remaining placenta can cause hemorrhage in the mother. I also had to inspect the cord to make sure it contained three blood vessels, since any other number is a sign of congenital anomalies. After this we inspected the vaginal canal for signs of trauma. In her case, as in many, the baby lacerated the vaginal wall into the perineum, the area between the vagina and anus, requiring me to help sew her up. Upon completion, I removed my gown and moon boots and went home to finish my ob/gyn clerkship. It was 11 PM and *my* "baby" was at home waiting up for me.

My rotation on ob/gyn was intense with long hours and awkward patient encounters. It was a good introduction into the surgical world. I definitely loved operating and felt myself being drawn towards the surgical subspecialties. I had only six more weeks to go before my surgical rotation. Time was running out for me to make a final decision on my career.

Chapter 8: Pediatrics

Slightly better hours than ob/gyn, my six-week pediatric rotation was next, the first three weeks in clinic from 8 AM to 5 PM. After that I did one week in the newborn nursery and two weeks on the pediatric floor of the hospital. During the inpatient rotation, I took care of the sick kids and learned a lot more than I expected. The pediatricians incorporated me well into their clinics. They allowed me see patients on my own, afterward presenting to them before we went in together. In other clinics that year I did a lot of shadowing and did not feel much like a third-year medical student. Being treated similarly to a resident was inspiring, something I needed as I neared fourth-year status and applications for residency.

During the outpatient weeks, I personally saw eighty patients and left with many of the diagnostic skills needed for pediatric clinic. The nursery week was quite slow for the majority of the time although I saw the similarity to the emergency room: slow one minute and frantically busy the next. After baby exams every morning, the attending and I would do "Mommy rounds" to let the parents know how their babies were doing. The rounds took place quite early since the babies always got farmed off to their mothers later in the day for feeding.

When the afternoons were slow, the residents took us to the Neonatal Intensive Care Unit (NICU). Unlike anything that I had envisioned since I had seen only adult ICUs, it housed to capacity rows and rows of tiny babies on ventilators. The residents picked out some of the interesting patients, and we examined them for whatever pertinent pathology they exhibited.

For instance, one had a loud heart murmur that we auscultated with our stethoscopes. Another baby in dire condition was very premature, having lived seven weeks on a ventilator that oscillated continuously, giving him tiny little rapid breaths. His whole body shook with each one, and I could only imagine the barotrauma being caused. He was grossly swollen and was fighting off infections, including an abscess near his liver.

One of the neonatologists paged us the following day for what we thought was slide review of certain diseases. When we arrived, however, he was gathering all of the residents and fellows in the NICU to head to the basement. When we walked into the autopsy room in the basement of Loyola, I saw the still, tiny body of the ventilator baby on the table, splayed open from the top of his chest down to his pelvis. We postulated theories for his death, canvassing his open organs for clues, and detected a yellow spot on his right lung. When the pathology resident asked me for my theory, I replied, "Infection," a hypothesis later confirmed when I saw the consolidation on the CXR taken before his death.

In babies, they strip the chest and abdominal viscera out in one large mass. After the pathologists had removed the organs, they began taking samples for histology. All that was left of the baby I had rounded on the day before was a head and body that looked like a deflated rubber suit, lying there until the neuropathologist arrived to remove the brain for study. Apparently there had been a major bleed in the brain that needed evaluation. Holding the baby's head over a bowl of water, he cut the skull along the sutures, producing a quick slide of the brain into the bowl. While a newborn's skull is quite soft, I was surprised at how soft the brain had become. The pathologist reported that the entire cerebellum had died from lack of oxygen because of an obvious blood clot. The brain's deterioration was a result, I believe, of a combination of the bleed and the weeks of being near death, yet we were able to keep the patient alive as long as we did through modern technology.

For me, this was a poignant moment, one that stayed with me throughout my day. I pondered the process of desensitization that seemed to be the norm in these situations. In fact, most of the residents who had been called away from their tasks at hand for the autopsy seemed mildly irritated to have been disturbed, some even leaving the autopsy early to resume their previous work. The only house staff that stayed the whole time with me was the neonatology fellow who had previously cared for this particular baby for many weeks, her primary interest to learn the cause of death so she could become a better physician. Afterward, we transitioned back into efficiency, even discussing lunch and the annoyance of being late to our noon conference.

The amount of callousness that occurs would shock most people outside of the medical field, but I am slowly learning that it is a survival mechanism that allows us to continue in a field where every day is someone else's worst day of life.

At the end of my week in the nursery I had to get up at 4:30 AM to round on the little ones with the team. Having lost one hour of sleep because of the time change, I was hoping to get out of there quickly; however, the most memorable baby of the week gave me quite a bit to think about. His young mother had confessed to her ob/gyn that she had been addicted to Vicodin right before delivering, having taken dozens of pills per day. We can usually take the number of pills an addict confesses to and multiply it by three to get a more accurate estimate. We could already see the effect on the baby: withdrawal symptoms of irritability and poor feeding and sleeping.

Vicodin is in the same family as morphine and heroin. Few birth defects occur as a result of their use but the withdrawal symptoms can be severe. Opiates cause a patient to relax, go to sleep, and feel no pain. Conversely, their withdrawal causes agitation, poor sleep, and autonomic disturbances such as changes in blood pressure and heart and respiratory rate.

We caused quite an uproar behind the scenes with the nursing staff when we allowed the mother to breastfeed for a few days. In fact, they were going behind our backs and complaining to their supervisors, but they didn't understand the physiology behind addiction. Having received a high amount of drug in utero, the baby's "supply" was now abruptly cut off with withdrawal symptoms appearing. Since a much lower amount is excreted into the mother's breast milk, breast-feeding could help the baby wean off the opiate without major symptoms. Furthermore, if the baby got any worse, we would give it morphine as a rescue therapy. And, of course, the breastfeeding could be allowed for only a few days, and then the mother would need to seek treatment for her addiction. Yet, to make matters worse, still living at home with her parents who were ignorant of the situation, she would not allow us to make it known to them. Our hands were tied with patient confidentiality, but we strongly advised her to explain this to them. We knew she would need strong social support, both for herself and her baby.

The final two weeks on inpatient pediatrics consisted of taking care of sick children admitted to the hospital. I personally cared for patients with hemorrhagic stroke in the brain, chronic pain, pneumonia, seizures, and intense vomiting from a narrowing in the GI tract. Other patients on my service ranged from a crippling genetic disease to child abuse.

Unfortunately, the young child with the genetic disease never left the hospital. He had a rare disorder that pretty much had disabled him from a young age, causing rapid body deterioration and requiring his mother to become a full-time aide. There was tension in the family because the father had the fight-to-the-very-end philosophy while the mother was exhausted and wanted to let him die in peace; not that she loved him any less.She just realized the futility in artificial prolongation of a life. This was not the first time he had been hospitalized, but, due to his deteriorating condition, it was likely his last.

One morning at 2 AM, I typed in the nearly two-page-long list of medications into the computer system. His mother, through trial and error, had developed most of the medical regimen, some of the medications completely unfamiliar to me. It was without a doubt the longest medication list I had ever seen. Every thirty minutes, 24 hours a day, medications had to be given through his feeding tube. This meant that the mother was constantly at his side unless she hired a nurse overnight. Quite frankly, I can understand her exhaustion.

The boy seemed lifeless as I looked at him. Ravaged by disease, he suffered from bloated and edematous skin, a common finding near death as the body loses the capacity to regulate fluid compartments. I felt sad for the entire family. I knew they were struggling to find a solution that offered no easy answer. Then, as if the situation remedied itself, the child died, circumventing a bad situation over how to care for him and uniting them in the grief of the child they loved so much.

I've always heard that losing a child is one of the most difficult things that can happen to someone, something hard for me to imagine since I did not have children at the time. Research shows that a child's death causes a strain on the marriage and life, in general, especially if a strong family bond doesn't already exist. Even though this family had a sad ending, the love the family had for one another made it less devastating and a sharp contrast to the next family.

On my last call night, a mother brought her three children to the hospital after they had been beaten up by their father. They had cuts and bruises but nothing serious that we could decipher from physical examination. We did skeletal surveys to be certain and found their injuries not to be life-threatening.

While the team was rounding the following morning, the mother's entrance provoked in me an immediate pity for the kids. Wearing dirty, ratty jeans, she walked about with her top pulled over her breasts exposing her entire belly. All I could see were tattoos, stretch marks, and flab. I was somewhat surprised that no one else seemed that concerned and continued with the work at hand. I kept expecting someone to say something, but I guess they had seen it all before.

The kids were so innocent, caring only about when they could go play. Here we had children seemingly oblivious to their woeful situation, with a drunken, abusive father and a mother with serious fashion issues. At least she appeared to care for them. I suppose that is all that one can hope for in a situation like this. As for the father, I have no sympathy for someone who could hurt his own children; hopefully, he was locked up with the key thrown away.

The most heart-wrenching patient was a young boy with severe scoliosis. We rounded on him every morning and each day he would be in tears from the pain. Having had multiple surgeries on his spine to try and correct his curvature, he unfortunately suffered many complications such as infection of the bones. Subsequently more operations were necessary to clean out the infected tissue and metal rods holding his bones together. Due to his chronic illness, he appeared extremely malnourished and tiny. The nurses told us he was so depressed he could hardly smile anymore. He should have had to worry only about what cartoon to watch on Saturday morning, not whether or not life was worth living in constant misery.

When checking on him each day, we set him up to examine his wounds, encouraging the nurses to do the same on a regular basis. It is just not healthy for anyone to be in bed all day without some movement. Yet, with each movement, he cried in pain, so the morning was not pleasant for any of us, least of all, the little boy. To make matters worse, his pregnant mother had been put on complete bed rest for the remainder of her term, so his depression worsened dramatically without his mother's comfort and nurturing touch. And I think we can all remember those times when we were young when only our mother's presence and comfort would do. After his cleanup surgery, he began to do better, but I knew it was going to be a long road of recovery for him.

Obviously, I was gung-ho about learning procedures and hands-on experience. When my resident learned this about me, he quickly taught me how to do nasopharyngeal cultures. The basic purpose is to get a sample of snot from the back of a squirming child's nose to test for a specific virus. Although this is not quite what I had in mind when I mentioned procedures, I did it with a smile and tried to help out as much as I could. Before any procedure can be executed, we must gather the materials, which can often be frustratingly difficult since only the nurses can get the materials from the cabinets, and they are usually busy doing something else. This procedure simply requires a bucket filled with ice for the specimen and a syringe with 1cc of clear saline.

Once the equipment is in hand we have to convince the patient that the procedure is not going to hurt, an episode that can range from a couple of seconds to a couple of minutes, give or take a few. No matter how convincing one is, an extra pair of hands is always needed to pin the patient down who always screams as if he or she is in the utmost agony. The sampling itself takes only a few seconds. After inserting the small tubing connected to the syringe about three inches into the nose, we quickly inject the saline and suck it back up. The syringe, full of snot, is then placed into the ice bucket and sent to pathology.

When word got around that I knew how to do the cultures, I began receiving requests from the other busy residents. Showing initiative and helping out residents will always come back to help in the long run. It wasn't long before the residents gave me more responsibility and attention.

Another interesting part of my pediatric rotation was Operation Homefront, a requirement of my rotation that involved visiting the family of a child with a severe handicap and seeing what life was like beyond the doors of the hospital. During my visit, I had the privilege of meeting an autistic boy. Six years old, he had experienced social, behavioral, and motor delays since birth. His brother also had autism but was at school during my afternoon visit. His mother was kind enough to invite me into her home to see what life was like in the day of an autistic boy.

She began the afternoon by talking about the different struggles she faced since the birth of her sons. Almost immediately following each birth, the mother expressed her concerns that something was wrong with the children, but no one listened to her. After a long delay and overdue diagnosis, her pediatrician apologized for the delay in diagnosis, explaining that he had only one lecture on autism in medical school. Thankfully, due to the increasing awareness and prevalence of the disorder, more emphasis is being placed on it in medical schools across the country.

Financial hardships accompany a diagnosis of autism, especially since many insurance companies will not cover the cost of private tutors and aides to help with developmental progression. Apparently aids charge as much as $100 per hour, which can easily cost upwards of $10,000 per year. The specific symptoms she described were diverse in nature. They ranged from the typical autistic symptoms of speech and fine motor delay to hypersensitivity of the senses, a peculiar anomaly present from birth in this child. If he tasted something new, he would immediately vomit, presenting a lack of variety in his diet. This was his mother's main concern because she wanted to make sure that he was getting enough nutrition. He also could not be in restaurants or large crowds such as birthday parties because the auditory distractions overwhelmed him.

After we had talked for a while, it was time for his bi-weekly therapy. His private speech therapist allowed me to shadow for one hour as she worked with him on many different skills. She intertwined educational games with eating lunch and got him to eat yogurt and a peanut butter and jelly sandwich, his mother reacting to the news as if she had won the lottery. These were brand new foods for him and good sources of fat and dairy that he did not previously have. It was interesting to see her reaction over what most people would consider a trivial event. This recapitulates what she said many times before the session: people with autism are wired differently and what we take for granted is sometimes a milestone for them.

Being in their home brought about a different perspective I never could have experienced in the clinic or hospital. This was a helpful reminder that behind every patient is much more than a diagnosis. With that, I left for my small break with great anticipation. It was finally time for my surgery rotation, and I entered it with a mixture of both excitement and dread.

Chapter 9: Surgery

The surgical rotation is the most difficult of third year in terms of hours worked and stamina needed to impress the attendings and residents. I placed this rotation at the end of third year because the surgery option was the last specialty I ever thought about going into. Two months of general surgery were followed by a month of two different electives, with the first month on the hepatobiliary/transplant service. Our attendings did general surgery with an emphasis on the liver until an organ became available for transplant.

Two other medical students and I had to split up the transplant cases since the month was a slow one in terms of transplants. Consequently, I scrubbed in on only one kidney transplant the entire month. Two teams worked the surgery, one team harvesting the kidney from the donor, a living relative, for her son while my team prepared the boy for the transplant.

Since the harvesting team began early, I sneaked in to see how it all worked. The surgeons used a laparoscopic technique to minimize the invasiveness of the procedure. One incision was larger than the rest so that the surgeon could squeeze his hand into the abdominal cavity. They inflated the belly with air to increase visibility, which caused the intestines to spill out of the larger incision. They feverishly tucked the intestines back until they could get a round, green gel seal with a centered hole in place over the incision. This hole stretched enough to accommodate the surgeon's hand but stopped just short of allowing the intestines from spilling out. The seal allowed the surgeons to also pierce through it with their equipment, which included tiny fiber optic cameras on flexible rods to visualize the anatomy.

When they were getting close to removing the kidney, my team went into the room next door and began opening up the boy. Normal kidneys are nestled below the ribs and toward the back, explaining the lower back pain in urinary tract infections. In the transplant procedure, the kidneys are retained in order to keep patient trauma to a minimum while the donor kidney is placed in the pelvis on the right side. When I asked why this is the case, the surgeon replied that it was simply convention.

When we were alerted that the donor's kidney had been harvested, we crossed back to the other room to prep it, careful not to touch anything as we were scrubbed in and sterile. After placing it in a bowl full of ice, we hooked it up to an IV.

Elevating the saline bag about 10 feet in the air allowed gravity to more efficiently pull down the fluid, doing so in order to flush out the mother's blood to decrease antigenicity. All that was left was to anastomose the artery, vein, and ureter to the recipient. The surgeons deftly executed the tiny sutures and knots necessary to prevent leakage of blood.

After we released the clamp, the kidney instantly turned from white to red as it was reperfused with blood. Thrilled to see the ureter almost immediately produce urine, the surgeon allowed the sterile urine to drain into the abdominal cavity. After connecting the ureter to the bladder, we closed up, and the job was complete.

Transplant surgery is quite exhilarating but comes at a cost for those dedicated enough to enter the field. The organs become available both day and night and do not care about schedule or sleep. The liver surgeon at Loyola had earlier postponed his vacation for a liver transplant and consequently missed a Cubs game. I definitely respect them for their sacrifice and dedication.

The first patient assigned to me was an ICU patient. Talk about tossing me into the deep end of the pool without as much as a life jacket. ICU patients are incredibly complicated to a young student with no critical-care experience. The middle-aged female patient had been admitted for overdose of Tylenol.

Apparently, she had been prescribed a potent Tylenol product for a recent outpatient surgery but took much more than she should have. Her liver began to shut down, and she became deathly ill in days. Since Tylenol is broken down by the liver, taking too much of it is extremely toxic. A biopsy showed greater than 80% necrosis, or death of the liver cells. Overnight, she was diagnosed with fulminant liver failure and moved to the top of the transplant list in the country. Each day I arrived an hour early to pre-round on her before the transplant team arrived. The numerous lines in her body made it difficult for me to keep them straight, emphasizing my inadequacy and requiring several questions for the medical residents covering the ICU. They were very accommodating in supplying me with the answers needed to complete my surgical notes.

The body's complex balance can tip when a traumatic event occurs. When a major organ such as the liver begins to shut down, many other organs will naturally follow. The first organs to follow suit were her kidneys, creating a condition known as hepato-renal syndrome, or kidney failure, caused by the liver. While we initiated dialysis to compensate for the slack in the filtration process by the damaged kidneys, the damage didn't end there. Her intracranial pressure began to rise to dramatic levels; much more of this and her brain would have squeezed out of her skull like jelly. In order to save her kidneys, she needed fluids, but too much fluid would increase her intracranial pressure even more and risk brain death. Such a delicate balance had to be managed carefully. To monitor the pressure in her skull better, we consulted the neurosurgery team to drill a bolt in her skull and place a monitor directly through the bone.

Each morning I read the residents' notes regarding the palpation of her expanded liver on physical exam. The liver is located underneath the rib cage on the right side. If one is a severe alcoholic, self-palpation of the enlarged liver is possible. For an alert patient's exam, he or she takes a deep breath as the diaphragm displaces the liver downward, subsequently brushing it against the doctor's hand. In a sedated patient such as mine, the best I could do was to wait for the ventilator to give another breath and palpate as well as I could. Although I tried my best, I never really felt it; I tried to convince myself that I had, but I never would have if I had not known from the notes that it was enlarged. This can be very disconcerting to a young medical student. If I couldn't feel the liver in a patient with fulminant liver failure, could I feel confident in my exam skills? Multiple times I asked the surgical residents to take five minutes to teach me how to find it, but I was never successful.

The arrival of the next suitable liver could occur at any moment, so we were all equipped with a pager at all times. The marathon of liver transplantation does not allow for sleep nor does it cancel the following day's schedule; otherwise, it would not be general surgery. Surprisingly, my patient began recovering from her symptoms, clinically improving little by little until she was taken off the transplant list. She still had to be slowly weaned off the ventilator and spent weeks in the hospital. All of this was the result of taking too much Tylenol, underscoring the seriousness of even the most commonly used over-the-counter medications. One physician said it best: "Every single medication should be regarded as a poison."

Although I am glad she didn't need to undergo a major, life-altering surgery, I ended up not getting to see a liver transplantation that month. Once again the dichotomy of training versus patient well-being rises to the surface. Although we students bemoaned missing the experience, a patient's well-being always wins in the end.

Most of the other surgeries I scrubbed in on were general surgery. One was a colon resection for colon cancer. This old guy was really nice, and I enjoyed rounding on him for the next few days in the hospital. I even saw him in clinic the next week, and it was interesting to see the continuity of care and the final results of all of the hard work. Whether or not he will survive depends on whether the cancer spread microscopically before we got to it. I also watched a guy's underarm skin be cut out due to a painful condition called hidradenitis suppurativa. In this condition, the sweat glands get chronically infected and need to be removed. We simply removed a portion of the skin and sutured the incision closed.

Some episodes in the OR were tenser than others. During one tumor removal, we cut into a major vein and blood began squirting out and filling the abdominal cavity, subsequently obstructing the surgeon's view. A few choice words were thrown about while he barked out orders for certain tools to stop the bleeding.

While the scrub tech searched in vain for the correct instrument, the tension in the room rose dramatically as the seconds seemed like hours and time began to slow. The tool was missing from the surgical kit, so others were substituted to do the job. Everything turned out fine, but it certainly gave me a little scare.

I had some great experiences that month, but I hoped to get more OR time in the next rotation. Both attendings took turns going on vacation, slowing things down considerably, even though the majority of time was not spent operating. We had to manage post-op patients for several days following their surgeries. We also acted as consultants for another service to give opinion on one of their patients, a most memorable patient with chronic hepatitis C and liver cancer.

A critically-ill, elderly Muslim patient, he was not the cheeriest of all patients, to say the least. He spent the entire month in the hospital so I saw him quite often. Each and every day I rounded on him in the early morning hours, long before sunrise, to check for an increase in jaundice (yellow color of skin) or ascites (fluid in the abdominal cavity). This was the patient case in which I finally learned to check the lines each morning to make sure they were in place. He had several lines in place for a variety of purposes, often pulling them out overnight because of delirium and sometimes just plain stubbornness. Not knowing about these developments would make me look pretty stupid on rounds, as the surgical chiefs expected me to know everything about my patients.

Although the transplant team tried as hard as possible to get him on the liver transplant list, he was just too sick and subsequently rejected, forcing him to wait for death. Every few days his distending belly was tapped and drained of a large amount of fluid. One early morning as I stood outside his door recording his vitals from overnight, I could hear his cries to Allah from the dark recesses of his room. He was in misery and there was nothing we could do other than supportive care.

After my completed month, I transferred to a different service. By chance, one day during my rounds in the intensive care unit, I saw him and noticed his obvious deterioration. A few months later I decided to type his name into the computer system to see what had happened to him. He had died a few weeks before. Just knowing that someone I cared for had passed away was sad, reminding me that despite all the medical advances, we are still remarkably limited.

As aforementioned, third-year level floor work is quite tedious, so the opportunity for hands-on action is quite exciting. One of the responsibilities that can be delved out to the third-years is the removal of staples on post-op patients. Since I had seen this done on ob/gyn, I assured my resident that I knew how to do it, proudly retrieving the proper equipment from the nurses when the chance arose. Similar to the desk-type staple remover, the medical version has two prongs that hook under the staple while one goes over it. Clamping down pops the staple out.

Sounds simple enough, right?

Wrong.

This poor lady had an incision spanning the entire length of her abdomen. To add insult to injury, she was a chronic pain patient with a litany of other problems. On the very first staple, I had the device flipped upside down, burying the staple in more tightly. She cried out in pain as I profusely apologized while trying my best to execute its removal. Everything I tried seemed to only make matters worse. I could see the area turning red as the skin began to tear. At one point she even got up to vomit. Needless to say, I felt terrible by this point so, after I quickly removed the 30 other staples, I left to get the intern. Of course he had to be at a table with dozens of people around to hear my little dilemma. Unfortunately, not even he could get the staple out, working and manipulating for at least 20 minutes. We finally had to order up special equipment to get it out.

Apparently, the staple had been manipulated into an "O" shape by so much handling. When we finally freed it, the patient was extremely and understandably relieved. I returned to the computer station to finish my note and proclaim my little incident to my classmates. They were going to hear about it anyway, so I figured it was best to hear from me. I was feeling humiliated until I recognized the lesson in it: although this was the first time I ever hurt a patient, it was likely the most insignificant by comparison, making me so much more aware of my responsibility for life in this field. If I felt this bad over an episode that was not life-threatening, how much more horrible would it be to be responsible for someone's death? I'm going to try and make sure I never have to know.

The second month of general surgery was a little more interesting with days easily lasting thirteen hours with some weekend work. I probably worked around 60-70 hours per week, not counting the hours of studying I had to cram into the picture. The only reason I didn't approach the 80-hour limit is because I didn't have to take call as much as the residents, whose generosity played a part, I'm sure.

Surgery is definitely a tough field, yet no other feeling compares to that feeling one has when scrubbed in with the surgeons under the hot lights. The surgeons on my service were colorectal, endocrine, and general in specialty. I witnessed a lot of neck surgery under the direction of the endocrine surgeon who, subsequently, was the leading expert in the region on endocrine pathology. He had subspecialized in thyroid and parathyroid removal. Although he was extremely hard on me, he taught me more than any attending had so far that year. His meticulous performance in every surgery made dangerous surgeries easy and without complication.

The morbidity from this type of neck surgery is damage to the recurrent laryngeal nerve. Approximately the size of a piece of thread, these two nerves run down each side of the neck, embedded in tissue and, consequently, are very difficult to find. A slip of the knife on one side can produce life-long hoarseness; if the other is cut, the patient's airway could close and cause death. As an aspiring ENT, I knew I wanted to perform these surgeries in my future practice so

I watched eagerly, absorbing every bit of information I could process.

During the operations, the surgeon often paused to ask me about respective anatomy or about the embryological derivation of the structures of the neck. For the most part, I answered his questions correctly and confidently, thankful for the previous warning from my colleagues to always be prepared for the Q & A. The worst thing I could do would be to answer his question with another question.

The parathyroid glands are tiny structures around the thyroid that are very difficult to identify. To make certain we were removing the right structures, we drew blood at the beginning of the operation in order to measure the level of its hormone, which breaks down rapidly. Consequently the blood sample had to be physically rushed to the pathology lab in the basement of the hospital, a glorious responsibility that fell to the third-year medical student.

After grabbing the sample, I sprinted to the locker room for my white coat and then hustled down the stairs to the lab. Since the blood was drawn in series, I often had a maximum of five minutes to run to the lab and return to the OR gowned up in the proper clothing. My record time was less than three minutes. I was proud of my new record, but it lasted only one day when an overzealous and competitive classmate defeated it by thirty seconds. Some may have considered it grunt work, but I didn't think it was so bad. We took turns so each student had to be a runner only a third of the time. The other two-thirds were spent operating on the fascinating neck anatomy that I loved.

While not as busy as the neck surgeries, the colorectal surgery was still a vital learning experience. We affectionately dubbed this service "the butt clinic" where even the residents became grossed out occasionally. The attending had a great sense of humor and joked along with us. Most of the physical exams involved putting a patient on an electrically powered chair, moving his or her butt into the air, and then sticking scopes, tubes, and fingers into the rectum to evaluate for cancer.

The surgeon taught me that the differential for a patient coming in with rectal pain is usually one of the following: anal fissure, thrombosed hemorrhoids, cancer, abscess, and trauma. Fissures and hemorrhoids can usually be fixed by incorporating more fiber into the diet, which makes the bowels regular and prevents straining. One patient on exam had an external, thrombosed hemorrhoid that looked like a giant scab. The physician took a paper towel and literally ripped it off. This apparently helps it to heal. I'm not so sure the patient appreciated the effort though.

Since fissures are not always visible, the way to tell if they are causing the pain is to touch the area with an instrument. If the patient nearly catapults off the table, the physician can rest assured the culprit is a fissure. Even though this clinic nauseated me at times, I hold those in the field in high regard. Medicine is such a great field since everyone can find a niche that matches personality and interests.

Interestingly, the colorectal surgeons can also perform colonoscopies. At this point in time I thought that GI specialists were the only doctors who performed them. The patients are put into a haze so that they are still awake but very groggy. If they do fall asleep at any time during the procedure, they rarely remember any of it. This is good, very good. Although this is not a comfortable procedure to undergo by any stretch of the imagination, and I do mean stretch, I highly recommend that everyone get a colonoscopy at the proper age.

After gowning up, we insert the flexible scope into the patient's anus and watch on the TV screen set up in front of us. Maneuvered through the winding path of the colon, or large intestine, this scope usually provokes moans and cries of pain as the scoping is the most uncomfortable part of the procedure. At this point, the patient would receive some more sleepy medicine and become quiet. Once the scope was positioned at the far end of the large intestine, the resident would slowly pull it back, rotating it with his controls to inspect every square centimeter of intestine. Clumps of slimy green "prep" could be seen everywhere.

The patient drinks the prep the day before in order to clean out the intestines of feces that would obscure our view and gross us out. While I was still grossed out, I was still impressed by the technology. Not only is a camera mounted on a scope that can be manipulated in three dimensions, but it also pumps air into the colon at the press of a button. This air is used to inflate the colon since it would otherwise collapse on the endoscope. It must, however, make its way back out at some point. Abnormally large expressions of air (farts) lace the atmosphere throughout the procedure.

At one colonoscopy I almost didn't gown up because there wasn't room for me to do anything. After standing at the foot of the bed in my shirt and tie for about ten minutes, one of the nurses asked me if I wanted a gown. I agreed and gowned up for the remainder of the procedure. Nearing the end of the procedure, I noticed a fine spray of feces and prep on my gown in spite of my distance from the table. I said a prayer of thanks and walked out with a smile.

I make light of the experiences I went through but colonoscopies are deadly serious. Colon cancer is perhaps the most preventable cancer in the world, but the second leading cause of cancer deaths in the US. Small, undetected polyps grow for a number of years before turning cancerous. If people would simply take the one day of embarrassment, tens of thousands of lives would be saved every year.

I came to realize that what my white coat did for my self-esteem wasn't always ironclad assurance for those on the gurney. Patients and their families constantly asked me my age, or, better yet, told me that I looked like a 13-year-old, these instances occurring most often in the ER and pre-op waiting room. I presume other patients thought the same thing in other situations but had the courage to ask my age only when they were seriously ill or being prepped for surgery. Imagine the emotional state of those being prepared for surgery and having a pip-squeak medical student informing them that he would be participating in their surgery. While most patients were very nice about it, others couldn't disguise the look of sheer panic on their faces.

One particular time epitomizes this ego-buster for me. During my introduction to a female pre-op patient, she exclaimed, "I told them I didn't want any medical students." Somewhat caught off guard by her abruptness, I informed her that her request could be granted with approval from the physician. Sometimes extra people are needed to retract tissue out of the way, whether they are medical student, resident, technician, or nurse. We do, however, try to put patients at ease and try to compromise with their wishes. I remarked that hers was a highly specialized procedure, so I wouldn't be scrubbing in anyway. Her insistence that I be nowhere near the operating room left me flustered and embarrassed, so I excused myself to talk to the resident.

When I found the chief resident in the OR, he was not amused whatsoever by her attitude. The camaraderie in the medical field protects the medical student's education. Granted, these same surgeons could bear down on me later for not knowing the answers to their questions, but that is part of the training process. He instructed me to stay because it was part of my education. I did so, and as she was being wheeled into the room, I feared she would spot me out of the crowd of people and make a scene. One of the scrub techs was, however, made aware of her concerns.

We decided to wait for the attending surgeon to arrive and run it by him before making a decision. This guy had a commanding and confident presence that earned respect from those of us training under him. All attention rested on him when the technician told him of the situation. He simply stated that since I wasn't scrubbing in, it wasn't a big deal. But, when the tech told the surgeon that the patient was adamant about my not even being in the room, he wasn't very happy, to say the least.

"You know what," he said raising his voice a bit. "This is a teaching institution, and if she doesn't like it she can go somewhere else!" The technician had her answer and gave me a little wink. Later the attending walked by me and gave me a reassuring pat on the shoulder, a significant gesture for a young medical student. People don't often realize the importance of these academic centers, where medical students must work for both knowledge and confidence. If all patients were like the previous uncompromising patient, kicking out medical students because of fear, a huge gap in training would prevent the best of health care. After all, some of the finest care in the world is delivered at academic centers, so we must be doing something right.

This episode interrupted the dynamics of our team. Usually the post-op patients were rounded on in the early morning hours to gather information and vitals to make team rounding quicker and easier. Because of her attitude, none of us were assigned to her, slowing us down on rounding. Yet, this was a great lesson. After that, I couldn't have cared less about attitude. If someone snapped at me, I was neither shocked nor upset, realizing that dealing with poor attitudes is just a hazard of the occupation, probably just like every other occupation out there. Similar occurrences happen all of the time at universities, but the majority of them are on the ob/gyn rotation where, in this day and age, most males expect it and are therefore not surprised when it happens.

Every Friday, we had teaching rounds with the attendings with everyone rounding on all patients on the service. The required rounding had already been performed early in the morning. The purpose of our Friday rounds was for the attendings to teach us practical information about real patients. Difficult questions were the standard routine; if we could not answer them in so many minutes, the questions were graduated to the senior residents.

We nervously prepared days in advance in order to know everything about our patients. A couple of times we were lucky and had only a few patients on service. Not that we didn't want to learn, because we did; we just felt a little intimidated by the process. In medicine, developing thick skin early on will save a medical student a lot of trouble. I was berated several times for not having a particular lab value memorized and ready to regurgitate to the attending. Each time I had to look in my notes for information, I expected repercussion for not being prompt in response.

Although the experience is not a comfortable one, we must realize that this is a serious business that leaves little room for mistake. Too often medical students float through rotations having been given no real responsibility. We complain about this often but then never seize real opportunity for responsibility when patients are assigned to us. If we don't make an effort to know about a critical lab value, then we deserve the reprimand. Although being under constant fire without encouragement would increase the already high levels of stress in the field, a designated teaching time once per week to push us to work harder is not too bad an idea. Most classmates of mine hated the surgery rotation because of how difficult the surgeons can be. Overall, I think a compromise could be struck between the two sides to provide a great learning environment coupled with high expectations.

Later that month in the OR, we were prepping a patient for surgery, and I was the only person in the room with the scrub techs and nurses. No resident. No attending. All of a sudden the patient sat up and started vomiting. We got her to lie down but things went downhill from here. She started convulsing uncontrollably and things started getting crazy. People were shouting and looking to me for answers for which I had none. They wanted to page the resident, but he was out of town and I had no idea which resident would fill in. We began to worry that since she was halfway sedated she might aspirate her vomit, which can be life threatening. With her shaking uncontrollably, someone ran to the side of the room and kicked a black button near the floor.

"CODE BLUE" rang out through the entire operating center. Seconds later the room filled with people and crash carts. The attending was close by and came into the room. Soon thereafter the trauma surgeon with his team burst in. He immediately asked for gloves and a knife and took over the situation, preparing to stick a tube through her neck right there to help her breathe. Although the patient calmed down, the surgery was cancelled. Still, what a rush! Luckily, the crisis was over almost as soon as it started. The Neurology consult wasn't sure whether or not it was a seizure. Most likely a drug reaction caused her to have difficulty breathing, from which she panicked with the lack of inhibitions caused by sedation.

My on-call experiences were equally exhilarating. On my first night the service was slow so I hung out with the trauma team with whom I responded to three traumas at once, including a young lady injured in a motor vehicle accident and two kids with falls. To the outsider, it seems like a chaotic scene but in reality, it is closer to controlled chaos. The injuries were serious but not enough to go to immediate surgery. They were each admitted for observation.

During my second night of call, I was reading in the conference room in the surgical ICU (SICU) when one of the residents came in and said someone was about to be coded. In the hospital, a code is called when a patient is on the verge of death and needs immediate intervention. I rushed into the ICU room where many people had already gathered. Each time we entered we had to gown and glove ourselves, because this particular patient had developed antibiotic resistant bacterial infections. We desperately tried to find a pulse since her blood pressure had dropped enough to be unreadable by the monitors, which pretty much indicates impending death. She coded a couple of times, and we brought her back with pressors and chest compressions. I observed with careful interest, knowing that before long I would be running codes myself.

One of the more senior residents called her husband and children to advise them of the serious nature of their family member. Some of them who lived in other states questioned the seriousness before making the long drive at night to Loyola. Since the patient had been sick for quite a while, they had undoubtedly had previous scares in which they thought she was close to death, so we reemphasized the bleak prognosis. Her body was so wasted from disease that she barely looked alive even before her death.

Earlier in the year, she had been admitted for hernia repair, plagued with complications ever since and subsequently ending up in the ICU. During one of the codes, a framed picture of her with her family caught my eye. She looked so young and full of health, a stark contrast from this ravaged body covered in bruises and discoloration from coagulopathy. Her lifeless eyes seeped mucus, staring at the ceiling, her body shaking with every breath from the ventilator. The awfulness of death was upon her, as she passed right before my eyes. The chief

81

called the time of death; most of us breathed a small sigh of relief. While we do not wish death upon anyone, we were relieved that her suffering was now over.

The field of medicine offers an amazing opportunity to save and extend lives. On the other hand, to everything there is a season, a time to let go and allow people to rest in peace. The patient's case was subsequently presented at a conference designed to improve patient care at Loyola. The complications that took her life were sad, but at the same time we in the medical profession have the humility and ambition to learn from our mistakes and become better doctors.

Just as the chief had called the patient's time of death, I felt my phone buzzing in my pocket. It was Nicole, and I called her later that night explaining why I didn't pick up earlier. As I talked to her on the seventh floor skyway of the hospital around 11PM, I took in the beautiful night skyline of Chicago. Amid the frenzy and work, there is a uniquely peaceful feeling in the hospital late at night. Reflecting over the events of the night made me so humble and proud to be in the field of medicine. Suddenly, a helicopter began its descent to the landing pad below. Throughout the hospital's loud speakers, "TRAUMA CODE YELLOW" alerted us to prepare for the incoming patient. I hurriedly got off the phone with Nicole and joined the residents in the trauma bay.

Soon the Flight-for-Life paramedics burst into the trauma bay carrying a 17-year-old boy with a stab wound to his abdomen. The wound was swollen and engorged with blood, protruding roughly two inches from his body like a giant knot. Blood poured out of the opening while we began our evaluation. We started the primary survey: the ABCs (checking airway, breathing, and circulation). Next, we checked the neurological status and exposed the patient's entire body to look for other wounds in the secondary survey. We got a stat chest X-ray and a FAST ultrasound of the abdomen to check for intra-abdominal bleeding.

The FAST is a quick assessment of the abdominal and thoracic cavity to check for signs of internal bleeding. He writhed in pain as we tried to get the name and number of his parents. Right behind him was his friend who had also been stabbed. I had no time to check on him to see how serious he was. Another resident began the same sequence of evaluation on him as our first patient. We then transported the patient to the OR for immediate exploratory surgery. The trauma attending was paged and an entire OR team was called.

This type of teamwork is seen only at Level 1 Trauma centers such as Loyola. I was surprised at how busy the OR was in the middle of the night. I soon heard that a lung transplant would be going on in the room next to us. The surgeon, chief resident, and I opened this young man's abdomen from sternum to pubic bone, exploring his entire GI tract by running the bowel to check for holes. Finding a hole in his diaphragm, we put a chest tube in to drain blood and secretions from his chest cavity. We also found lacerations to his stomach and sewed them up. Initially, I would have expected a lacerated spleen since its anatomical position warranted a hit, but he was actually very fortunate that nothing else was damaged. A spleen laceration can quickly cause death since it is highly vascularized.

The operation was soon over, and I went to the call room to try and get a few hours of sleep. I was paged at 4:30 AM to scrub in on an emergent appendectomy. The surgeon was so rough on the resident that I heard her crying at the end of the surgery. It bears repeating: the field of surgery is very tough. At this point in time, dawn was breaking, and it was time to get to work for the day.

I rounded on my patients in a half-daze from the lack of sleep. The daily routine of rounding as a team with the chief resident took place afterwards. I then scrubbed in on a parathyroid surgery and went to colorectal clinic before finally going home on hour 30. Ask Nicole how grumpy and tired I was that day! After sleeping for five hours, I got up to eat dinner since I hadn't eaten that day. After I watched two hours of TV, I went to bed and slept the whole night away. Such is the life of a doctor in training, and I wouldn't trade it for the world.

Chapter 10: Surgical Electives

My last month of surgery was an elective month with two weeks on peripheral vascular and two weeks on Otolaryngology (ENT). Since the final exam was only a month away, I hoped for some easier hours. Working a 13-hour day and then trying to read at the coffee shop is not easy. Peripheral vascular turned out to be some of the longest hours yet so my exam study had to wait. Still the rotation had some huge payoffs.

First of all, my chief was an amazing person to learn under, making me feel more like a part of the team than any chief had yet. Granted, I was the only medical student on a smaller service, so there was much more room to maneuver. I believe it was more than that though. Even if I may not have learned a lot of book knowledge, watching the way he talked to patients and delivered bad news was invaluable. In vascular territory, we have very sick patients we coin "vasculopaths" with terrible arteries to the point that their limbs rot off while still on their bodies. We try as hard as we can to revascularize them, but it is not always possible.

The different approaches to this problem depend on the situation. If a patient comes in with an acute clot cutting off blood supply, the first intervention is usually angioplasty. Similar to stenting the arteries of the heart during a heart attack, we can stent the arteries to the legs in an embolic or thrombotic occlusion. Thrombotic means a clot formed at a specific site and occluded the vessel. Embolic means a clot was produced elsewhere in the body, such as the heart, and was thrown down river where it clogged a narrower artery. If too much time elapses after the oxygen supply is choked off, the tissue begins to die.

We had a woman come in with severe pain in her entire leg. She had waited days before going to the hospital, partly because she was unable to walk and partly because she didn't want to burden her caregivers. While I can attest to the honest attempts at salvaging her leg through angioplasty, it was no use. By the next morning her right leg had turned black. I used Doppler to try and find a pulse somewhere in her foot. At one point, I remember getting excited about palpating a pulse only to realize it was my own reverberating through my fingers. I was present as the chief broke the news to her that she was going to lose her leg. She cried as he held her hand with an empathy I was not used to seeing on a surgery service. At that moment, the impact of two months of general surgery took its toll on me. Grueling hours and the constant barrage of pain and suffering made me retreat psychologically in order to avoid dealing with the stress. I was further sickened when I recalled the callous joke I had told another resident about the "little leg that could." Simply put, I am not proud of those moments.

It was my chief that reminded me what medicine is all about. Another family became irate when they learned that their mother was going to lose her leg as well. Because of her heart problem, surgery had been postponed, yet no one had taken the time to explain the delay to the family. My chief patiently explained the situation to them, apologizing for their situation and repeating himself two or three times when necessary. Before we left that hospital room, the family was laughing about how they had overreacted. The chief taught me about the type of surgeon I want to be.

I witnessed a few rather intriguing surgeries on that rotation, the first being a carotid endarterectomy. The carotid is the main artery in the neck that feeds the brain. This patient's artery was nearly occluded with plaque. After clamping the artery through an open neck incision, we spliced it open and removed the giant plaque all in one piece. The plaque was so hard we could remove it without it crumbling. In the meantime, a plastic tube bypassed blood from one end of the artery to the other to keep blood flowing to the brain. Granted, there was another carotid artery on his right side, but no one knew how good his collateral circulation was. Since even the tiniest pieces of plaque could post-operatively embolize to his brain and cause a stroke, we carefully cleaned the artery of every speck. After placing a graft to widen the diameter of the vessel, we sewed him up and the case was over.

In the situation of a leg clot that has not caused the tissue to die, a bypass procedure can be performed. In one patient, a clot formed in the main artery of the leg around the level of the knee. We opened up her thigh and cut the artery after clamping it. I watched in amazement as the vascular surgeon attached it to the nearby vein. We then opened her up below the knee and attached the vein back to the artery. The clot was effectively bypassed and the perfusion to the foot preserved. It's astonishing to me that God made our bodies with so much reserve that we can perform these types of surgeries.

Concluding the major operations of those two weeks, the last case I want to mention was repair of an abdominal aortic aneurysm. Past procedures cut a large and painful incision in the belly to manually repair the largest artery in the body. We have now developed the technological means to repair it with only two small incisions in the groin, an endovascular procedure not unlike angioplasty of the heart. Under fluoroscopic guidance, the grafts are placed into the correct position as we all watch on the monitors. If discovered in time, a formerly lethal disease is now managed operatively.

That Friday my wife and I left for a weekend getaway to Lake Geneva for our one-year anniversary. I returned on Monday for my long-awaited rotation in ENT, the area I had all but decided to enter as a career. On day one I went to the OR in the morning with the department chair, a nasal and sinus specialist with referrals from all around the country. He was a very nice guy who answered a lot of questions I had about the specialty.

The first patient's nose was almost completely occluded from nasal polyps. I watched with interest as the specialist guided one of the chief residents through the entire case. They passed a scope with a mounted camera through the deep recesses of the face. Equipped with a red light easily visible through the patient's skin, the endoscope had a chewing device that destroyed the polyps and simultaneously suctioned them out.

Following the moving red light, I watched the scope pass the eyes and enter the forehead. During his clinic in the afternoon, I had the chance to see many surgical patients for follow-up. Many had suffered from chronic sinusitis or other conditions that severely affected their breathing and sense of smell. It was exciting to see how thankful they were just to be able to breathe again.

The following day was spent with a pediatric specialist. The OR schedule was stacked with tubes, tonsils, and adenoids, all very quick procedures. The entire procedure for ear tubes takes less than ten minutes. Under the microscope, a small incision is made in the eardrum and the tiny tube is inserted.

The procedure for tonsil removal is also easy. Located in the back of the throat on each side on the mouth, the tonsils have to be cut out manually with electrocautery to minimize bleeding. The indications for removal are multiple sore throat infections per year and large size obstructing breathing.

The adenoids, on the other hand, are slightly trickier. They are located in the very back of the nose, requiring them to be removed through the mouth blindly. A probe with a looped blade is positioned right behind the uvula, the "punching bag" hanging down in the back of the mouth, and scooped vigorously removing a large chunk of bloody tissue that subsequently releases a torrent of blood that has to be cauterized with the bovie. The bovie uses electrical current to fry the bleeding vessels. This may seem harsh, but it is still a quick procedure with little risk.

The next physician I rotated with was a head and neck cancer specialist. The first case was a bilateral neck dissection to remove cancerous lymph nodes in a patient with melanoma. We started by making an incision below one ear, curving all the way down the neck, and then up to the ear on the other side. I retracted the skin flap as the residents freed it up to the jaw to expose the entire neck. We then began the process of lymph node removal along with any salivary glands that looked cancerous. We made our way all the way down to the jugular vein and meticulously cleaned off the fascia. At one point we could see a muscle that attaches to the shoulder blade, highlighting how far in we had to go. Four of us including the attending had scrubbed into the operation, so there were a lot of hands in close proximity.

I was at the patient's head retracting while the surgeon cut away fascia when it happened. I suddenly felt the raw sting of pain radiating from my left thumb as the surgeon's scalpel flicked passed. Time stood still as I held my breath, staring at the white latex gloves, praying that the scalpel had not penetrated my skin. Before long, however, red contrasted with the stark white glove as my blood begin pouring out of the laceration caused by a bloody, contaminated scalpel. "You got me," I replied, still in disbelief. "Scrub out!" a resident proclaimed. I hurriedly pulled off my gown and gloves while I heard background orders being barked by the attending physician to get a bottle of betadine or alcohol.

I rushed over to the sink and began scrubbing the wound. An OR tech came over and poured an entire bottle of alcohol over it while I scrubbed for nearly ten minutes in the sink. Thoughts of HIV and hepatitis began floating through my head. Who is this patient? Is he high risk? I hadn't met him before the operation so I had no idea who he was or where he had been. While no doubt his blood entered into my wound, the actual rates of transmission of HIV and hepatitis with needle sticks are rather low, which was some comfort to me.

However, this was no needle stick; it was instead a tiny laceration that bled heavily for at least ten minutes. I remember thinking that the one hundred dollars I paid the previous year for the hepatitis B vaccine now seemed like a good investment. The maniacal thought of HIV and hepatitis C reminded me of my previous patient with terminal liver cancer caused by chronic hepatitis C infection.

By the time I entered the OR again, the patient's blood had already been sent off to the lab for source testing. They sent me down to the ER to get blood drawn myself. One of the nurses in Fast-Track told me I had to be triaged like everyone else in the ER. I sat for nearly an hour in the waiting room in my scrubs and white coat. Imagine the number of stares I got: a medical student with a bloody cloth wrapped around his thumb and reading a book. Not that I minded waiting like everyone else; it was just a little embarrassing to be the center of attention like that.

When the triage nurse finally called my name, she seemed stunned to see someone in scrubs. She advised me never to wait like that again and to come right up to the triage station. I later learned that these blood draws are generally done immediately without any waiting time. This policy helps to minimize the anxiety involved in such a situation.

After I got into the Fast-Track department, they took a baseline blood draw for me to help with reimbursement in case I seroconverted to HIV or hep C positive. I waited only a couple of hours before the rapid HIV test came back negative.

What a relief! I now found it safe to call my wife to let her know what was going on. We had to wait only a couple of days for the hep C serology of the patient to come back negative. Only then did I begin to feel relaxed. Such is the occupational risk of being a surgeon. I have had numerous needle sticks since then. It is inevitable when you work around sharp instruments day after day.

Almost everyone around the operating table had his or her own story of being cut or poked by a contaminated instrument. In a way, I actually felt inducted into a surgery club of sorts, even receiving a much-coveted apology from the attending. He was high up in the ENT department, so I banked on some definite sympathy voting come application time. Well, not really, but it couldn't hurt to dream a little.

After my little scare I jumped right back into the fray to forbid the incident from scaring me away from surgery. The next cancer case was a woman with melanoma on her scalp. We excised a piece of scalp about the size of a baseball all the way down to the skull. Such a large margin is necessary due to the lethality of melanoma after it invades the dermis (skin). To check for metastasis, we injected methylene blue dye and radioactive particles into the lesion before the operation. We then used a sensor to locate the first lymph node the radioactive particles drained to. It was located right below the angle of the jaw on the left side.

After cutting into the skin, we saw the blue-colored lymph node. Removing it for pathological examination, we then traded out with the plastic surgeons to close the large open lesion on her head. Plastic surgeons specialize in skin flaps and often team up with other surgeons in order to cosmetically reconstruct or close wounds that cancer surgeons have created. Since I had worked from 7AM- 5PM without so much as sitting, eating, or using the restroom, I decided not to stay. I really wanted to see the closure, but I figured I would probably do a plastics rotation at some point.

One morning we began the day with a simple tracheostomy, a usually quick procedure of inserting a breathing apparatus directly through an open incision in the neck. Sometimes, these procedures can even be done at bedside if the patient cannot be moved. Since sick patients in the ICU are often ventilated for weeks at a time, a trach allows them to be more comfortable. Still, having a breathing tube down the throat is no holiday.

That morning the residents began the surgery while the attending was in another OR. Since we anticipated a quick procedure while awaiting the next case, I didn't even scrub at first.

About fifteen minutes into the case, the chief told me to go ahead and scrub, which I thought was a little strange at first. Assuming he felt guilty about my not getting in on the action, I scrubbed up and returned to gown up. I entered an atmosphere thick with tension. The chief needed me at the head of the patient to help retract the tiny incision, so I took my place right in the way of the anesthesiologists who were trying to manage the patient's airway during the surgery. When the airway goes, so does the patient. From this vantage point, I could see everything, including the cause of the delay.

The patient's thyroid gland was directly in the way and had to be split in two. Often the thyroid can be bypassed with the tube inserted directly above or below it. The thyroid is highly vascular and fiercely bleeds when not properly cauterized. Additionally, it is difficult to use the bovie that close to the airway. Hot flame immediately juxtaposed to concentrated oxygen could cause a small explosion that would burn the trachea and lungs.

Blood began to fill the incision faster than we could suction it out. At one point we entered the airway and blood began leaking into the lungs. The residents fiercely sutured the thyroid trying to achieve hemostasis. To make matters worse, we didn't even transfer the patient from his ICU bed into an OR bed. For the entire case we were slightly bent over, as the bed was wider than the typical bedding used by the operating rooms. This made it more difficult to see, and our backs began to ache and fatigue. Time was now against us as the clock ran past forty-five minutes.

At one point the resident began shouting, "Suction!" but the intern could not see well enough to suction properly. "I can see!" I shouted as I grabbed the instrument from his hand and quickly suctioned the blood. It spurted out of the traumatized gland almost as quickly as I could remove it. Now, I need to explain the repercussion of what just happened here. A medical student never takes anything out of the hands of someone his senior. While no one said anything, the situation had obviously justified the action. Still, I was worried about it for a while.

Finally, the attending walked into the room and asked if we needed help. We accepted the offer, and the operation was over within ten minutes. What a difference the hands of experience make.

I then began to explore the subspecialties of ENT I still had not seen during my third-year rotation. Among these were otology (ear) and laryngology (voice/airway). The otologists are ENT-trained physicians who do one to two years of fellowship afterward to perform deep ear, skull-based operations. Among these are cochlear implants and removal of acoustic neuromas, tumors of the inner ear only millimeters away from brain tissue. I also saw reconstruction of the middle ear on patients with distorted anatomy from previous tumor removal. The tumor of the middle ear cavity is called a cholesteatoma. Technically, it is more of a skin appendage than a tumor and grows from the eardrum into nearby skull. All of the surgeries otologists perform are under a microscope due to the tiny anatomy. They usually go through the back of the ear, cutting and retracting it out of the way. They then chip away at the mastoid bone, the skull right behind the ear. "Chip away" is probably too loose a term; drilling better suits the scenario.

The laryngologist I worked with focused almost entirely on disorders of the voice box. Keep in mind a general otolaryngologist rarely sees this much of any one subspecialty. Difficult cases in each category are sent to centers such as Loyola where subspecialists reside. Since he focused on voice, he had many singers and radio broadcasters that traveled to see him. After each office visit, we performed a procedure by sticking a scope down the patient's nose or mouth to get an up close and personal view of the vocal cords. Sometimes we found nodules or signs of cancer. Other times we would find only symptoms of gastroesophageal reflux disease, which usually manifests itself by swelling and redness. For most patients coming in for voice changes, reflux was the culprit. Luckily, this is easily treated with antacids.

My brief stint in ENT during third year was enough for me to make the decision to pursue it. I learned two things that year that forever changed my life. I wanted to be a specialist, and I wanted to be a surgeon. Although this had been my preliminary decision, I wanted to know for sure by going through the day to day routines. I like the variety of ENT. For instance, I can see children with ear infections and senior citizens with cancer. I can perform a variety of surgeries in one day encompassing traditional "open" surgery, microscopes, and endoscopes. I also have the option of doing a fellowship and focusing in on one area. This would narrow my focus and allow me to become a leader in the niche of my choice.

After third year, I had a week off to relax and run errands. Basically, I had a week to get my life back in order in preparation for the fourth-year marathon. I had originally assumed that fourth-year hours would be more merciful, but I was in for some surprises.

I was also apprehensive about the whole residency application process, which would require a lot of traveling around the region for interviews, if I were lucky enough to get them. All of this, however, was something that was going to have to wait until after my break.

Chapter 11: Fourth Year: The Electives

Fourth year of medical school is composed primarily of electives chosen by the students to best prepare them for their specific specialty. Neurology, ICU, and Wards (the latter two known as sub-internships or sub-I's) basically taught us how to behave like interns, who are essentially in their first year of residency and are the workhorses of the hospital. They generally work the longest hours, executing most of the grunt work the senior residents don't want to do.

Quite frankly, the intern assumes the kind of responsibility that can be costly to the patient if a mistake is made, such as being one decimal off in a medication order at 2 AM. For this reason, we spent a substantial portion of our time fine-tuning medical knowledge and mastering simple but significant details, such as how to put orders into the computer system.

Although fourth year offered rotation through specialties that I will probably never practice, I learned skills that will prove invaluable in my chosen field. Set up a few months in advance, each rotation was a month-long, creating a rolling schedule that allowed me to decide what to rotate through as I went along. This schedule allowed discretionary time (code for vacation) in which I was able to take a month off in December to do residency interviews, study for Step 2 of the boards, and spend time with my wife. Planning for discretionary time at the end of the year allowed me to not only finish a month early but also to make preparations for my transition into residency when decompressing is most necessary. Besides, this was probably the last time in my life I would have such a large chunk of time off.

By comparison to previous years, fourth year may be easy, but it still entails the aforementioned difficult rotations as well as the process of applying to and interviewing at multiple residencies. The stress of applying to a competitive residency is exacerbated by the financial strain of traveling across the country and interviewing at programs while trying to subsist on the small number of loans given. I think it's safe to say that Nicole and I lived rather modestly during my medical training. We were by no means poor, but half of our resources coming in were high-priced loans gaining interest every day.

I also had to balance the responsibilities of multiple research projects. While my cardiovascular surgery project was coming to a close after two years of work, I also had ENT research projects competing for my time. Since having published research is a great application builder and talking point during interviews, I was in a race early in the year to get these projects published. Deadlines approach quickly: applications for residency began in the early fall; interviewing season came in the late fall/early winter.

Rotations, research, and applications to residency also had to be balanced with the responsibilities of teaching the Patient Centered Medicine course for the second years. My last-minute decision to help teach this course to the younger students allowed me to "give back" as well as earn two extra weeks of vacation. I showed up for a few afternoons here and there and taught the second-years how to do pertinent clinical tasks such as write-ups for the physical exam. Although they were learning how to do the complete physical exam throughout the year, they also needed to know the medical abbreviations to summarize the results.

I volunteered for any sessions that had to do with the head and neck. The passion for one's own specialty becomes apparent and facilitates in teaching. After answering questions and teaching the students the detailed write-up, I took them to a clinical room where they practiced the physical exam steps covered that day in lecture. After they observed my single demonstration, they, in turn, would practice while I observed them to check their progress. Because this actually benefited me as much as it did them, I highly recommend to other medical students to find some way to teach younger students at their respective schools.

All students usually begin the year in their specialty of choice, which includes a rotation at a different university to audition their talent and knowledge. I began with ENT, followed by my surgical ICU month, after which I felt so much more competent and that much closer to becoming a physician.

Chapter 12: Otolaryngology: Head & Neck Surgery

Every medical student in the country schedules the specialty he or she wants to go into early in the summer of fourth year, basically to audition to the attendings, residents, and staff members for a residency position. Just knowing that the slightest mistake could cost a residency spot at a particular institution is often overwhelmingly nerve racking.

My two-month block in ENT was undoubtedly the most important in my medical school career. Generally, my best-laid plan was to do a home rotation before venturing away to another program. Before doing a clinical month, I performed a month of research with the Chair of Otolaryngology, a sinus specialist, collecting data on all of his surgery patients from previous years.

My task, sorting through all of the charts and placing the collected data into an Excel spreadsheet was a monumental task. Having been asked to provide a review paper to a journal with worldwide circulation, the sinus specialist offered me the opportunity to compose it, which I gladly accepted, realizing the advantages of a department chair's support.

My clinical month was divided between the gold team, red team and the Hines Veteran's Hospital (VA). The gold team consisted of pediatrics and ear. The pediatrics rotation focused on bread-and-butter tubes, tonsils, and adenoids common in this population. Because these surgeries can be slightly trickier in very young children, these sub-specialists are often needed, especially for the highly dangerous surgeries on neonates. These premature infants often spend an extended time on a ventilator, causing a narrowing of their airways which, in turn, can lead to respiratory distress and often death. The ENTs can remove these lesions or dilate them with a balloon.

The ear specialists perform a variety of surgeries ranging from skull base tumors to clean-up operations in people with terrible ear infections. This subspecialty is quite competitive for obvious reasons. Restoring someone's hearing is a very gratifying experience. The skull base operations are also very interesting, as this involves removing tumors deep inside the skull with drills under a microscope. Surgeries like this are often comprised of teams of neurosurgeons and ENTs.

On my first morning at around 6 AM, I paged the resident, who was already rounding in the pediatric ICU. I joined the rounds on a young female patient with cerebral palsy, admitted with respiratory distress. Having been trached, she was struggling to breathe, coughing through the hole in her neck. I remember inwardly cringing at the sight and thought of a young child suffering, thinking "I don't like this."

Suddenly, a large ball of mucous blew out of the hole and splattered the shield covering the trach tube. Immediately, she relaxed in her bed. "There you go," the resident told her comfortingly. We rounded on her every day that week, checking her airway to make sure it was open and checking the tubing. Her breathing difficulty put things into perspective; coughing up some phlegm never posed a life-threatening situation for me. For this young child it required a tremendous effort. Until that moment of relief came, she suffered from silent suffocation.

I applaud the thousands of parents who deal with this type of caregiving. Some people have put their own careers and personal pursuits aside to focus on the higher priority of caring for a special-needs child. It is the truest form of unconditional love. While the general public may believe that they get nothing in return for their love and devotion, I believe that they reap a gamut of reward for their dedication.

Other patients we saw on gold team included a temporal bone cancer of complex quality and another trach patient. The former was going to be discharged without a definitive cure for her ailment. Because the site of her cancer was the temporal bone, the skull plate behind the ear, she was under the care of the ear specialist. As with the young patient with the breathing difficulty, the only other patient on our service at the time had a trach tube placed for airway problems. The surgical process of placing a tracheotomy tube in the neck creates a permanent hole in the midline of the neck for airway access. The tube can be capped when a patient is feeling better and opened at night or when he or she is having respiratory difficulties. The hole in the neck needs a good seal in order to produce enough airway pressure to make sound.

When I first saw the adult patient, she couldn't speak because of the tube's improper size. Immediately after the problem was corrected and the tube capped, she was able to talk again. True, she sounded a bit like Minnie Mouse, but she could talk, much to her joy and relief. At that moment, I began to experience the exhilaration of helping patients as an ENT. Since most of the senses such as hearing, taste, smell, and voice are in the head, I will be able to help restore these abilities to anyone who has had to live without them for any period of time. And, although the eyes fall under the ophthalmologist territory, ENTs operate in the periorbital region in cases of abscess or cellulitis, so I may be able to help restore someone's sight. With this in mind, one can understand how competitive the field of otolaryngology is and what a reward it is to help restore someone's ability to hear, taste, smell, or talk again.

After rounding, I spent the first two days of the week in clinic. Day one was with an ear doctor while day two was with a pediatrics doctor. Clinic isn't nearly as exciting as surgery, but it is where medicine is learned best because of the opportunity to follow up with the attending about the management of each patient. Since ENT is highly specialized, I shadowed in the clinic, which is something I didn't enjoy. I needed to supplement the medical school teaching of ENT pathology with more depth and detail.

I spent the first day of the week with one of the most highly sub-specialized ear surgeons in the country. Ironically, I had a raging ear infection from swimming at a resort in Wisconsin the previous weekend. I felt embarrassed to bring up my own health concerns on the first day of service, but by noon I was in too much pain not to say anything. Reprimanding me for not speaking up earlier, he put a special cocktail of drops in my ear that would kill anything. He also gave me a prescription so I didn't have to schedule an appointment on my own. Finally, after my financial investment in the medical community, I was getting some perks.

I think the most interesting patients seen that day were BAHA patients. Bone anchored hearing aids are devices implanted in the skull behind the ear in certain patients. This new technology is improving the quality of life for many patients with hearing loss. Unfortunately, at Loyola, I didn't get to see placement of any of these devices or cochlear implants, which are hearing devices implanted deeply in the inner ear. General ENTs can't perform cochlear implants without an ear fellowship: Otology, Neurotology and Skull base fellowship to be exact.

The girl with BAHA I saw that day came to clinic with her mother because of a technical problem. For some reason, part of the device outside of the skin had broken off, creating the need to re-implant the device under anesthesia. We were somewhat taken aback when the mother began weeping, but realizing why she was crying didn't take long. She had lost her health insurance and currently couldn't afford it. Apparently, she had a job lined up and might get insurance in the near future, but, in the meantime, the child would have to go without.

Seeing an innocent child affected by the insurance quagmire we have in this country was distressing. It's quite a dilemma we have before us. Driven by capitalism, the advances catapulting this mind-boggling technology boom in medicine must be financed somehow, somewhere, by someone. Without it we would be back to the dark ages of medicine. Luckily, this young girl will likely not have to wait long to get her medical care.

In Tuesday's clinic with the pediatric specialist, I saw a multitude of young children with ear infections and obstructive sleep apnea. This specialist's repeated prodding for questions caused me to think constantly in every patient encounter for scientific questions. For one thing, I would have zoned out halfway through each visit if I were no more than a nuisance in the corner of the room. He introduced me to every patient, had me look in every ear with the otoscope, and, most importantly, he tested my exam skills by asking me about the eardrums he had just inspected. The ear exam is not easily mastered, so I was glad to have learned much more than if I had simply shadowed him. I didn't leave there a master at clinical skills, but I did leave with improvement. Ending my clinic days on gold, I anticipated three interesting surgical days.

Two of the days were with the pediatric specialist. The vast majority of the surgeries consisted of ear tubes, tonsillectomies, and adenoidectomies. Now that the specialists knew that I had declared the field of ENT, I received more "attention to detail" surgical training, even though I didn't get to do anything. I soaked up every bit of detail I could because I would soon be doing these surgeries myself.

The specialist's management of surgical days was a wonder to behold. Working between two rooms, he performed quick operations while teaching both the resident and me. I already had compiled a mental list of questions for him if he asked for them. Fortunately for me, when he asked the resident if I had asked her any good questions in his absence, she was able to answer in the affirmative. He was testing me to see if my questions were simply for show and not true intellectual curiosity.

A couple of interesting cases of direct laryngoscopy and bronchoscopy, fancy terms for looking down the throat, presented themselves for my repertoire of learning. Usually the patient is a trached child who has developed a stenosis in the airway due to trauma or inflammation. If a child with a trach develops respiratory distress, a DL&B is needed to rule out a narrowing. We had balloon catheters waiting in the rooms in case a stenosis was found. I had carried the very tall packages over from the hospital since they weren't available in the outpatient OR, receiving a number of stares since they were almost as tall as I. Finding no stenosis in the children, we simply changed the trach tubes.

I was a little surprised by how hard the ENT residents worked even with the absence of pre-rounding. Each day I either quickly grabbed lunch whenever I could or I didn't eat at all. Rounding around 6:30 AM each day was the norm, except Wednesday, which was at 5:30 due to morning conference. This is earlier than I had to round on my general surgery rotations, which many students complain are the longest hours of any specialty.

The conferences on Wednesday enabled a developed camaraderie among us, made even better by the attendance of both attendings and residents. The morning generally began with lectures to continue the learning process, all of which were very stimulating to me because of the newness of the material. More and more I liked the idea of being a specialist with knowledge and skills that most in the medical community don't have. Giving up a lot of general knowledge for the specialized information was a better trade.

Following the lectures, oncologists and radiation oncologists specializing in head and neck cancer met with us for the tumor board joint discussions on the current cancer patients at Loyola and Hines VA. Naturally, while otolaryngologists are surgery-biased, the oncologists are chemo/radiation-biased, thus creating a debate environment that is fascinating to observe. An ENT resident presents the patient along with any radiographic films followed by intense discussions debating the management of the patient. An attending may say something like "the recent literature states that patients with T2N1M0 squamous cell carcinoma of the oral cavity should be treated with surgery followed by adjuvant chemotherapy." Then their discussion started with the other attendings in the room either agreeing or disagreeing with support from their own research.

Post-conference we all scurried to clinic or the operating room. Unfortunately, I had only one day with the otologists in the OR. Time did not allow for further observation of some of the major skull and inner ear operations. During my first two years of medical school, I never thought I would be interested in ear surgery; but, after having witnessed the otologists' incredible surgeries, I am more convinced than ever.

The first surgical patient was a young girl with chronic ear infections, infections so bad that they had spread into the mastoid bone behind the ear. Comprised of air cells, this bone can become infected and fill with fluid, detectable on CT scan.

After draping the patient, the resident pulled up the microscope and began injecting local into the ear canal and behind the ear. Next, a C-shaped incision was made behind the right ear, which was then cut back and pushed forward toward the face and out of the way. While the ear appeared to have been removed, the result was a large, gaping hole where the ear should have been.

In order for all in the room to observe these procedures, students could use either a side arm on the microscope or watch the projection on the monitors. Technically, I didn't have to look through the microscope, but I wanted the practice. The bony ear canal could be seen in the middle where the eardrum resided. A square piece of fascia was removed and placed under hot lights to dry out, to be used later as a graft to reconstruct the eardrum. A chisel-like device scraped muscle and other tissue from the bone in order to expose the skull.

In one hand, the resident used a small pea-sized drill on the tip of a handle to bore out the mastoid bone. With the other hand she used a device that sprayed jets of water and suctioned at the same time, resulting in a shower of fine bone particles and water vapor. The bone was pulverized into millions of little pieces and suctioned out as a solution. The resident drilled at a very slow and tedious pace to avoid entering the brain. Every so often she would ask for a diamond drill, encrusted with microscopic jagged diamonds, to smooth the surface of the skull in order to clarify her work.

As the resident maneuvered the drill through the skull, she pointed out landmarks. In one area the skull began to change color indicating that a large dural sinus was only millimeters away and an area to avoid. Entering into this would cause a large hemorrhage. Another dangerous location is the skull base because of its close proximity to the brain. The last site of avoidance is a bony ridge containing the facial nerve. Damaging this nerve would cause facial paralysis.

The middle ear was carefully reconstructed and the fascial graft put into place to serve as a new eardrum. By the end of the surgery I was certainly convinced of its seriousness. By the time the resident was finished, under the supervision of the attending, the mastoid bone had been drilled and aerated. The ear was successfully ventilated and hopefully would not get any more infections. I could hardly wait for my opportunity to perform a mastoidectomy.

The next surgery I watched that day was fairly comparable except for its label of radical mastoidectomy. A radical procedure meant that less would be preserved due to the seriousness of the disease process. I watched tediously for hours as the resident drilled away at the skull until the attending finally came in to check on her work. "Uh oh," was the first thing he said when he looked through the microscope. "I hope she had a dead ear before surgery because she sure has one now!" the attending proclaimed.

"No, she could hear out of that ear," the resident responded. Suddenly the once boisterous room became chillingly silent as everyone wondered if the resident just ruined a person's hearing for life. The attending quickly grafted the delicate structures to protect them from further harm. An hour of awkwardness passed before the surgery was over. The resident was silent afterwards as we brought the patient to post-op recovery. The difficulty with surgeries such as this one is the fact that many of them are revision surgeries, follow-ups on someone else's surgery without knowing what he or she did or what scar tissue would be present. Tertiary centers like Loyola often get difficult revision surgeries because specialists are needed to fix the problem.

After the patient was awake enough to talk, we went to speak with her. Her ear was bandaged well so it would not be possible to test her hearing at that moment. However, we could use our instruments to determine if the ear was in fact dead. A tuning fork was made to vibrate and placed on the top of her skull. We asked her in which ear she heard the vibration. She responded with the right ear indicating that the ear still had some function. I could see the tension literally drain from the resident's face.

A person with normal hearing should hear, equally in either ear, a tuning fork placed on top his head. Someone with conduction hearing loss will hear the vibration more loudly in the bad ear. However, if the ear were completely dead, the sound switches over to the other ear. Therefore, although she had conduction hearing loss, this matched her situation before surgery. The entire situation was a real wake-up call for me: it is quite easy to ruin someone's hearing permanently, a difficult situation to deal with if it ever happens.

Overall, the gold team was an amazing, fast-paced week during which I definitely worked my share of hours. What was most interesting to me was the structure of the team: the junior residents took most of the pediatric cases and the seniors took the ears. At this point in the game, my first mastoidectomy would be a few years in the future, but, since I liked the pediatric cases as well, it wouldn't be a problem.

I spent the weekend recuperating and readied myself for the following week on the red team, which would probably be the longest hours of the rotation.

The red team consisted of head and neck cancer surgery, comprising a difficult week with long hours and poignant patient encounters. I definitely worked longer and harder that week than I did on my general surgery rotations, averaging around twelve to fourteen hours per day. We typically began rounding at 5:30-6:15 AM before heading to the OR or clinic. Head and neck cancer is definitely an interest to me, but the morbid surgeries are something to consider.

During rounds the first day the team went to see the patients on our list, the first becoming quite a stand-out memory for me. Entering the room, I noticed a sitter in the room watching him, but this is a common occurrence so I barely acknowledged him. The patient was a frail, elderly man with a trach in his neck. We weren't his primary service but were consulted on him to check his trach and see if it needed changing. The poor guy hacked and coughed while trying desperately to catch his breath. Every now and then he would blow the mucous out of the hole in his neck, nearly splattering us as we tried to examine him.

I couldn't help but feel sorry for him as he struggled to breathe. Who wouldn't feel mercy for him? As we prepared to leave, one of the residents began talking to the sitter, who revealed that he was not a security guard but a police officer. "Is he under arrest or something?" the resident asked. "Yes, for homicide," the officer responded. "He shot and killed his friend yesterday over a game of cards." We were stunned, to say the least. We all wondered how a guy so frail could be a cold-blooded murderer. The murder had occurred the day before, which was also a little alarming. Apparently, he had chest pain while in jail and was transferred under police supervision.

Having a murderer on our service was depressing enough, but the next patient was an attempted suicide. We rounded on her the entire week, but she was too sick for us to do anything for her. The prognosis was grim.

The clinics were mainly in the cancer center with a brand new head and neck cancer surgeon. He had done his residency at Loyola, leaving for one year to do a fellowship in tumor debulking and reconstruction. Because there is not enough experience in the five-year otolaryngology residency to do the major cases, a fellowship is needed along with a career in academia where residents can help round on the sick ICU patients on nights and weekends.On the first OR day I could barely wait to get into the OR. This is the type of surgery that wows everyone who sees or hears about it. In fact, even the heart surgeon with whom I was doing research enjoyed hearing about the cases.

The first was an inferior maxillectomy for recurrent cancer. The maxillary sinus is an open space in the cheekbone. The best way to access this without mutilating the face is through the mouth. The surgeon cut open the hard palate, otherwise known as the roof of the mouth, providing good access to the sinus. He then used a drill to bore through the bony structures, finding the necessity of removing some teeth in the process. I struggled to get a good view as quite a few residents were scrubbed in to witness it for themselves.

The large hole in the roof of the patient's mouth then had to be reconstructed. While the attending finished the debulking of the sinus, the chief resident and a junior began making a skin graft from the patient's thigh. A device that looked like a cheese slicer was rolled over the skin, producing a thin layer that curled away from the slicer. The resulting blood permeated through the damaged dermis, creating a strawberry-like appearance of the skin. The harvested skin was sutured into place in the sinus and the area tightly packed. Finally, a prosthesis temporarily replacing the bony palate was screwed into place.

Since the cancer was extensive, a neck dissection was needed, adding another couple of hours onto an already long surgery that had started around noon. The surgeons made me leave around 8 PM since I had been standing all day without a good view. They operated for at least another hour or two. After a week in the ICU the patient was healing nicely. We scheduled a follow-up visit with an oral surgeon who would place a more permanent prosthesis. Because this was the seventh surgery to rid the patient of cancer, we all hoped he would see success and that this procedure would be his last.

When there was no clinic or operating in the afternoon, an ample supply of consults awaited, proving again the rigorous schedule of a resident. On one occasion, I tagged along to see a patient who had thoracic surgery to repair an aortic aneurysm. Upon awakening in the ICU, he experienced hoarseness that did not resolve. Consequently, ENT was consulted to evaluate him. The resident asked me if I had ever scoped someone on my own. I hadn't and was delighted when he assigned the procedure to me.

After we interviewed the patient to learn more about his situation, we sprayed numbing medicine in his nostril and I readied the equipment.

The scope is a tiny, flexible fiber-optic tube with a camera mounted on the end. The tip can be adjusted up or down with a control on the handle to allow a snake-like movement through the nose to the back of the throat. Initially I maneuvered slowly, careful not to cause a nosebleed or unnecessary pain. When I arrived at the back of the nose, I instructed him take a large sniff to get past obstructing tissue. When that didn't work, I asked him to stick out his tongue, immediately getting a nice view of his vocal cords. To test their function I had him say "EEEE" in different pitches while I watched. I was so focused I didn't hear anyone enter the room. A family member who had arrived saw the tube down the poor guy's nose. "So much for that nap!" he joked before turning around and walking right back out the door.

I returned my attention to the exam, and the diagnosis was quite clear. The right vocal cord moved and vibrated while the left remained still. During his surgery, the recurrent laryngeal nerve on the left side had been damaged. Since the nerve wraps around the aorta, it is prone to disturbance. I had read in the operative note that the aneurysm involved this area so the nerve might have been stretched or cut in the repair. If it were completely cut, the guy could be hoarse for the rest of his life. Only time will tell. We referred him to the voice specialist at Loyola for follow-up care. There are procedures that can be performed later on to help with the voice problems. All I know is that I did my first scope and made a diagnosis at the same time.

The final operative day on the red team was a memorable one to say the least. I scrubbed in on the most morbid, incredible surgery I had ever witnessed. Remember, there is a weird dichotomy with the surgeon-in-training regarding empathy for our patients and excitement at a new and difficult case. The patient had a cancer in his nose that was misdiagnosed and neglected for far too long. It began ulcerating through the outside of the nostril. We planned to take off part of the nose but wouldn't know how much until we got in there.

The attending cut about a centimeter around the right side of the nose and down the left side of the nose along the midline to spare the left nostril. The idea was to use the left nostril as a flap to cover the large defect. From the get-go, things seemed to go badly. In the first incision in the left nostril, we could see tumor invading through the tissue. Therefore, a larger incision was needed to remove more tissue. Before long, the entire nose had to be cut off. A small surgery had turned into a life-altering event.

Unfortunately, the massacre didn't stop there. As we scraped off tissue, we saw that cancer had burrowed through the bones of the face. We had to break out the drills and bone crunchers. First to go was the right maxillary sinus. Next, we cut tissue off as closely as we could to the right eye without penetrating it. "I don't want to take the eye," the attending said. For one thing it would be unethical to remove someone's eye without proper consent. Second, it would probably be better to give radiation therapy a chance before ruining someone's vision.

Sadly, it did not end there. We had to go deeper and deeper into the face until a baseball-sized hole was visible where the nose used to be. Even the residents caught my attention with the "oh my" facial expression. When scrub technicians who spend their lives in the operating room are floored with amazement, you know something serious is going on. I could literally put my fingers all of the way into this hole. No one felt good about the situation. We felt sorry for him. However, the surgery had to go on.

At one point I had to trade spots with one of the residents who had no eye protection. A few minutes later the drill hit a pocket of blood, sending a shower of blood from the hole. Everyone standing around the table was splashed with blood, including my face shield. If the resident had been standing there, he would have been exposed to the patient's blood. In fact, he still got splattered on the face even though he was a few spots down the table. Although he wasn't splattered in the eyes, I made a mental check at that time to never get lazy and to always wear eye protection. It only takes one mistake to get infected.

A flurry of margin sampling unlike anything I had ever seen took place. Taking margins means to sample the borders of tissue and then rush them to the pathologists for a quick assessment of cancer spread. A sample would be labeled something like "right anterior inferior maxillary sinus mucosa." Over thirty-five samples were prepared in an all out attempt to save this man's life.

A few of the margins came back with invasion, and we debulked more in that area until they came back clean. With surgery finally over, all that was left was recovery. I think the patient handled it well considering the situation. He was comforted by the fact that a prosthesis could be made to hide the defect and give the appearance of a new nose. I hear they look quite real. The hope was that he would be completely cancer-free after a round of radiation to rid any microscopic cells that may have been left behind.

The last surgery of the week was a joint effort with the general surgeons for esophageal cancer. The entire esophagus, or food pipe, had to be removed. Our part was pretty small. We simply made access through the neck to get to the esophagus. When I walked into the room, the patient's abdomen was already split open. The surgeons' arms were bloodstained all the way up the elbows as they reached deep in the abdomen to cut out the esophagus. It was quite a scene to see both the stomach and neck opened up with large incisions. After it was cut in the neck it was easily removed. Sadly, the prognosis for this type of cancer is not very good. The patient was only in his 40's.

That wraps up the week with the red team. The main learning point was that the ENT residency is no walk in the park. The hours are very long on the cancer service. Some surgeries are ten to fifteen hour marathons with little to no breaks. In fact, the day of the nose removal, I had no meal breaks and didn't eat until I got home that evening. These sick patients must also be looked after no matter if it is weekend or holiday, which translates into little time off when on such a service. One day off per week is usually allowed but cannot be guaranteed. It is a sacrifice that one must make when entering a surgical field.

My week at Hines Veteran's Hospital was a culture shock to say the least. It took me about a day to get used to the differences between a veteran's hospital and a private hospital. First, the facilities are not as nice. The hospital was old and appeared run down at times. The equipment seemed older and getting through the place was like winding through a difficult maze. Surprisingly, this feeling of being in a different country fades away quickly and it becomes just a different building.

On the first day, we hit the OR all day performing minor procedures. One such procedure was a vocal cord nodule removal. The patient was obviously hoarse as we wheeled him into the operating room. He was a jovial guy, talking endlessly about his niece who couldn't make it there to be with him. Laughingly, he told us how he teased her about being on vacation while he was dying on the operating table. Of course, we all laughed since it was a simple procedure removing a harmless vocal cord nodule. We see these nodules all the time, and removing them is no big deal to the trained Otolaryngologist.

After passing a rigid scope through the mouth, the chief resident used a microscope to guide himself through the process of cutting the nodule out of the delicate vocal cord. One small slip of the knife and this patient could have been hoarse for life. He first cut into the mass and slowly peeled it away deliberately and meticulously. While the attending could have done it much more quickly, he instead guided the resident from behind. After all, this was a teaching hospital. With the surgery over, I forgot about the whole thing and went about my week.

Unfortunately, the benign-appearing nodule came back from pathology as cancer. The patient therefore had a regimen of debulking surgery, chemotherapy, or radiation coming his way. He could very well lose his entire voice box and never speak normally again.

Later that day we had a simple tonsillectomy on an adult patient. The senior resident quickly whipped out one of the tonsils. The junior then got his first chance to do a tonsillectomy. The five-minute procedure quickly turned into twenty as the resident struggled to stay within the fascial plane. A slight veering outside this area caused a lot of bleeding that took time to coagulate. Nothing serious happened but as I watched, I realized that I could be in the same situation in two short years. I found myself getting a little impatient after only fifteen minutes.

The next couple of days were in clinic at the VA. The vets are an interesting group to care for indeed. Everywhere on the walls are "Support the troops" posters as well as portraits of our Commander-in-Chief. Many of our vets are plagued with mental health problems such as depression and post-traumatic stress disorder. Social ills also plague them. Once, as I walked by the cafeteria in the basement of the building, I heard a commotion. I peeked in to see an elderly man seated in the back, cursing and screaming at the top of his lungs. Whether he was screaming at someone in particular or a figment of his imagination I do not know. What I do recognize, however, is that these people are heroes, because their sacrifice has allowed me to live on the safe side of war.

In that same cafeteria, a day later, I was eating with my fellow residents when another resident walked in. As she approached us, I noticed a dark, red rash around her neck. She and some residents commented back and forth about how she was doing well and healing nicely. After she left, I asked what had happened to her. Needless to say, I was shocked when I learned that she had been attacked by a mentally ill patient.

Apparently, someone walked into one of the clinics after hours and found her on the ground being strangled by a patient. This was a wake-up call for all of us to take precautions when working in certain areas, especially the psychiatric ward.

Overall, I must admit that the vets are a joy to care for. Most of them are extremely respectful patients that consider lowly medical students their doctors. Trivial statements to some are a big deal to a novice medical student desperately trying to become a competent physician. Throughout the week I noticed myself becoming more and more comfortable in my role there. I saw patients and completely worked up their plan for treatment before presenting to the doc. I was often wrong, but I learned from my mistakes and remembered them the next time they arose.

Social problems such as smoking and alcohol are a big problem with the vets. This combination is a recipe for disaster, cooking up all kinds of head and neck cancer. This is where the ENTs come in. Entire clinics were designated to care for the endless number of cancer patients. Some arrived with only bionic voices to help them speak, as their original voice box had been cut out via a total laryngectomy.

One big surprise was that residents could see patients without an attending. An attending had to be at the clinic to answer questions, of course, but the residents had the opportunity to begin developing confidence in themselves as doctors. I suppose I shouldn't have been too surprised.

Many residents in other specialties have clinics of their own. I got to see patients as well but then presented to the attending afterward. The attending would go in and double-check my work. I loved focusing only on the head and neck and not the entire body. That is the reason why I have a specialist mindset and not one of a general practitioner.

Perhaps the most interesting patient of the week was a young guy in his 40s who presented with a neck mass. He was also a paranoid schizophrenic, which is important when deciding about surgery and post-op care. A needle biopsy of the enlarged lymph node just below his jaw proved it to be a squamous cell cancer. This type of cancer never originates in the lymph nodes of the neck. The tonsils, tongue, and larynx are all common primary sites of origin.

One can easily see the need to find the primary site for a potential cure. Just cutting out the lymph nodes through a neck surgery would do nothing for life span otherwise. As often is the case, however, no primary could be found in physical exam or imaging. The best option for a difficult case such as this is a long, tedious surgery with multiple biopsies followed by a modified radical neck dissection. We got a late start with him since he wasn't taken to the pre-op holding area on time. The 7:30 AM start quickly became more like 8:30.

The first step was to get a serious look into this guy's throat. Imagine introducing a large metal, hollow rod into the mouth and all the way down the throat in the search for tumor. We did this and many other procedures in pursuit of the evasive cancer cells. A biopsy needed to be taken from the back of the nose. A small rod with a fiber-optic camera, along with a biopsy instrument with teeth, had to be guided through the nose. He had a very narrow passageway so it took a long time. Then, the nose began to bleed and the passageway quickly became obscured with blood and mucous. We finally got the sample and sent it as a frozen, meaning it would be read within the hour. It came back ambiguous.

Next, we set our sights on the tonsils. The junior resident got another chance to shine as he began the tonsillectomy. He struggled once again getting millimeters out of the fascial plane into the muscle. This caused bleeding which prolonged the surgery even more. The higher-ranked senior resident stepped in and had the second one out in minutes. After the biopsy steps were finished, we began the neck dissection, sending the specimens for permanent pathology with return in about a week.

About this time we heard weather reports about a major storm system making its way through Chicago. Rumors of tornadoes in the area also began to surface, making everyone a little nervous, especially when the hospital cordoned everyone off. Because we were in the basement of a gigantic building, I worried very little about myself. Most of all, I wondered if my wife would be able to get home safely from work.

Once we were ready to begin the neck dissection, a situation emerged. The cardiovascular surgeons next door were performing an esophagectomy for esophageal cancer and replacing it with the colon. They quickly ran into problems when they realized they couldn't proceed without removing the larynx, or voice box. The guy's colon was already out so they had to proceed. They needed an ENT but our attending was the only one available. The attending had to leave us right in the middle of our operation.

The senior resident was a brand new fourth year still getting comfortable with the leadership role. I could see the uneasiness in his eyes as we slowly entered the neck, trying with great difficulty to avoid the high priced real estate. Our painstaking efforts to be safe extended the time of the operation by hours. Luckily, a chief resident was available to come and assist us. A chief is a fifth year resident fully versed in nearly all ENT operations. Most of fifth year is needed only for developing confidence and racking up numbers of cases. They generally know how to perform most operations with great skill.

The attending darted back and forth when available since she worried about us. Seeing an intelligent resident years ahead of me in training still nervous about what to do was another reminder of how far I still had to go. He was four academic years my senior and until that moment seemed all knowing. Chiefs often appear this way to students. We know they are not perfect, but we still admire and respect them. As I was reflecting on this in the OR, I recalled a conversation with him I had had on the first day. I asked him if he was enjoying being "acting chief" as a fourth-year resident. "It's stressful" was his simple reply. "Well, you know we lost someone earlier."

He wasn't long into his senior status before one of the ENT patients died. I wasn't around when it happened, but I did hear about it. I could see the heavy burden in his eyes during that original conversation. I saw the same eyes that day in the operating room with the patient's life before us. It's remarkable how it takes events such as these to remind a medical student how serious becoming a doctor is. Of course, we all know what a great responsibility it is, but seeing it in action and feeling it is much different than reading or hearing about it.

The surgery ended around 5:30 PM and, by that time, the storm was raging. I stopped briefly in the break room to hear the news reports of collapsed buildings and dozens of injuries. I quickly called my wife, finding her safely at home but scared.

Work for the day was not over though: another small surgery still needed to be performed. A patient needed a tracheostomy but wasn't even brought down to the basement yet. I think the staff was hoping we would cancel the case so everyone could go home. No such luck since we are surgeons and don't cancel cases because it's late.

The residents and I took the elevator up to the 13th floor to wheel the patient down ourselves. The window outside was a non-stop display of lightning. We unhooked him from the ventilator and manually bagged him during transport. "Bagging" allows us to breathe for a patient in transport by squeezing a bag of air directly into their lungs through the endotracheal tube. After we made our way to the basement, we quickly got everything ready, put the patient to sleep, and were seconds away from making the neck incision.

All of a sudden...darkness! The power went out in the entire building. Imagine being in the basement of a building about to begin surgery in sheer blackness. The lights suddenly reappeared to our relief, but then flickered out again. The power outages didn't last long, but it was enough to end the case. I guess there *are* things out there that can cause surgeons to cancel surgeries. We wheeled the patient back to his room. We would have to get him tubed the following day.

After rounding on our patients, we called it a day. Arriving home after 8:30 PM, I ate the reheated remnants of dinner and went to sleep. I had to get up before five in the morning.

Luckily, the last day of the week was a simple half-day clinic. One quite memorable patient was a very elderly man with poor hygiene, reeking of cigarette smoke and body odor, whose personality outweighed the sensory onslaught. He had a history of skin cancer over his right temple area, the grapefruit-sized area having previously been removed with a skin graft sutured over the remaining defect. He was presenting for his routine follow-up a year later, answering my questions about his history during the physical. The paper-thin skin graft had left a very obvious brown spot on his face, while bony protuberances of his skull were quite visible. Though cosmetically deplorable, it got the job done. After I presented him a clean bill of health to the attending, the attending went in to see him for himself.

Right off the bat, the attending asked the patient about his apparent weight loss. The guy couldn't have weighed more than 100 pounds, a cardinal sign of cancer. Noticing that the rough brown edge of the skin graft was spreading outward, he brought in the chief resident who also appeared concerned about its appearance. It was clearly advancing over his eye. I was kicking myself at this time for not being observant enough. The resident and I then performed a biopsy of the area, but the brown crust seemed to flake off, revealing normal-looking skin underneath. If it were cancer, the skin below would have been invaded. Although we sent the biopsy to be on the safe side, what we were witnessing was a simple case of poor hygiene. Brown material had hardened over time to form a crust that had looked suspicious. We de-waxed his completely impacted ear canals before he left. Admittedly, this is not the most glamorous part of the specialty, but every field has its gross parts. If general surgeons can deal with the rectum, I suppose I can deal with earwax. Week three was now over and only sinus was left. I enjoyed learning the VA system even though it was shocking at first. My last day at Hines was also the first day I got off early so I enjoyed the small break while it lasted. The last week would be with the department chairman, and a great impression was crucial. Applications to residency were well under way at this time. Adding this to the research I was trying to get done on the side made for a stressful and busy time in my life.

The sinus week was relatively laid back. The other sinus/skull base specialist was vacationing, which created a much-needed break after the first three weeks on service. Despite the easier hours, the week was nerve-racking because I needed to make a good impression with the top dog at Loyola. On top of this, I had to finish my residency applications and two research projects while asking for letters of recommendation.

My first case was a middle-aged female with a painful mass in her left maxillary sinus. Radiographically, it had been diagnosed as a fibrous dysplasia of the bone, an apparently rare disease that is relatively benign. The best course of management was to perform a Caldwell-Luc procedure, an old-school surgical option used to operate on the maxilla, or cheekbone. An incision is made underneath the upper lip and the mucosa lifted until the maxilla is visible. This procedure has largely been replaced by the less invasive endoscopic surgery.

The bone is drilled out with a diamond bur with careful attention to the sinuses, nerves, and eye. A few millimeters off course with the drill could cause serious complications. A computer is used to help guide the process along. Simply sticking a probe into the area of interest will show where that location is on a large CT scan image, greatly reducing any possibility of damaging any sensitive areas and confirming complete removal of the diseased bone. I was completely fascinated with the procedure. Cool technology and a powerful drill, what more could a guy want? With the combination of rarity with both the disease and the operation used to treat it, I decided to do a presentation on the case in front of the entire department. I added this on top of the previously mentioned responsibilities I had to do that week. It was well worth the effort. After extensive research, I learned a lot about a disease I will most certainly come across later in my practice. Putting hours of work into one disease hopefully means it will not be forgotten.

The bread-and-butter sinus surgery consists of endoscopic surgery using scopes and drills to open up closed sinuses. The most common indication is a chronic sinus infection that is resistant to medical therapy. I did, however, get the chance to see a newer technique used to open the sinuses. A balloon was snaked over a wire guided into the sinus. Similar to angioplasty of narrowed arteries in the heart, the balloon was inflated to open up the narrowed sinus, a simple and straightforward procedure. I believe we will see more of this as technology develops and advances. Perhaps someday it will always be the first option, reserving conventional drills for balloon failures.

The next couple of days consisted of clinic with not too much excitement. I did, however, obtain my two remaining letters of recommendation and had good talks with the attendings, one of whom promised me his full support. His word carried a lot of weight in the academic world, so he gave me a lot of confidence in my chances of matching. Furthermore, one of the papers I wrote was submitted and accepted intoan otolaryngology journal with worldwide circulation. Having my name next to the chairman's name in such a journal was great for my application. The chips seemed to be falling into place.

The final day on service was interesting, to say the least. The younger sinus surgeon came back from vacation and had two interesting surgical cases lined up, the first one lasting all day. We teamed up with the neurosurgeons to remove a tumor on the pituitary gland, an endocrine organ that sits in a saddle of skull base called the sella turcica. The best way to get access to the deep recesses of the skull is endoscopically via the nose. The guy afflicted with this tumor had the typical double vision symptoms as the tumor began pushing on the optic nerves.

Having the latest and most up-to-date training and surgical skills, both the attendings were fresh out of their respective residency training and gung-ho regarding surgical challenges.

Their interaction was intriguing; they asked each other questions, teaching each other techniques they had mastered. Because access was needed to the skull base, ENT went first, using knowledge of scopes and small tools needed to debride far behind the face. Chippers and drills delicately cut away the deep membranes of the sinuses allowing the brain surgeon to work. Deftly punching into the paper-thin bone and reaching the brain, he removed the pituitary tumor over the course of hours. Images of the tumor on CT scan were pulled up on the large computer screens to help guide them. I missed part of their work, as we had to step out to perform a quick operation on another patient. Surgeons often balance multiple operations with the help of residents and other surgeons, such as the neurosurgeons in this case.

The other patient had sleep apnea and terrible snoring. We quickly cut out his tonsils, uvula, and soft palate. These structures comprise the room of the back part of the mouth. We sutured what remained to the sides of the mouth to hold the airway open. He had a severe sore throat for two weeks after that but his snoring remarkably improved. In addition, improvements to sleep apnea can improve overall health. The hour-long operation was quickly over, and the resident and I rushed to get back to the pituitary case. After we transported the awakened patient to the post-operative recovery room, we threw our masks back on and rejoined the neurosurgeons.

They were about to finish by this time. The newly created defect into the brain had to be closed to prevent bacteria from causing meningitis, a potentially life-threatening complication. A piece of fat was cut out of the patient's abdomen and placed into the hole. A flap created at the beginning of the case from sinus wall was then placed over the fat pad. Instead of completely cutting out the back of the sinuses, a small strip of fascia was left connected to a stump, keeping the graft alive via a blood supply.

Finally, the surgeons sprayed a green liquid over the entire area, which hardened within seconds to form a gelatinous seal. They felt confident that these three layers would be strong enough to keep the brain from herniating through the hole and, conversely, keeping pathogens out. To be sure, we put in a lumbar drain to lower the pressure of the spinal fluid around the brain. A resident inserted a large needle about four inches long into the patient's back. Next, he threaded a catheter into the area around the spinal cord to drain fluid.

I was completely exhausted by the end of the day. Not having a chance to use the restroom or eat all day didn't help. Although it was a challenging day, I thought it was appropriate to end my ENT rotation on such an exciting case. The teamwork of different specialties in the OR amazed me the most. I had heard of ENTs and neurosurgeons teaming up due to our close boundaries. Each specialty brings unique gifts and talents to the operating room. Inner ear skull base tumors are another area of teamwork between the two specialties.

Overall, I concluded my rotation with amazement and respect for the specialty. I was confident that I made the right decision to specialize in a field in which I can see hands-on, immediate results to pathological problems. Admittedly, I was surprised at how hard the residency is with long hours and few days off. It would be a difficult five years, but I knew I could do it. What helps the most is the camaraderie among the residents. They are all going through the same thing and develop a unique relationship with each other. I hoped to experience the same bond over the next five years of my life.

Chapter 13: Externship

A couple of months later I performed an ENT externship at the University of Illinois at Chicago's program. Most medical students do an audition rotation to check out a key program they are interested in. I spent the first morning running around an unfamiliar campus completing the appropriate documentation. Soon after, I was thrust into the OR on a monster case that had already begun, having no idea who was who or the particulars of the case.

The one thing I could ascertain was that it was a major neck dissection. Another fourth year was scrubbed into the case and two third years from UIC were watching. At first I couldn't really see anything, but, at one point, the field of view became clear. All of a sudden they pulled the tongue out through the neck incision; I was completely mesmerized. I hadn't seen an operation like this at Loyola.

It turned out to be a floor of mouth cancer that had invaded the surrounding tissue. After the tongue was removed and the neck dissected, the plastic surgery team came in and began removing a large, rectangular flap of skin from the patient's arm. The graft was then meticulously sewn into the wound and folded into the shape of a new tongue. An artery and vein from the arm were left attached to the skin flap and connected to an artery and vein in the neck. The necessary training to debulk large tumors and reconstruct the face with free flaps is executed in a year-long fellowship after the ENT residency.

Consequently, the chief resident was excited about this case because she wanted to do a fellowship in free flaps. For the next few days on rounds we used a Doppler to see if the artery was still working appropriately, placing it on the newly created tongue that protruded from the patient's mouth. Because the case had started early in the morning and lasted until midnight, I was sent home a little early because of the difficulty seeing through the crowd of people. Standing all day without operating made me inpatient for my turn with the knife.

Overall, the first couple of days at UIC were strange for me because everything seemed different from Loyola. At first, I had the stranger-in-a-foreign-land feeling, but by the end of the first week, I was having a great time. The residents were really into teaching, and I learned a great deal. Everyone dictated notes in clinic instead of typing; therefore, as a sub-intern, I was expected to dictate as well, which was surprisingly intimidating at first. I had never audio-recorded myself, so my first attempt was terrible. I'm certain the attendings had to thoroughly edit the final notes typed by the technicians. Still, it was a great learning experience for residency.

The next interesting case was a parotidectomy, a case I had wanted to scrub in on for months but never had the opportunity. The parotid gland is a salivary gland on the side of the face just in front of the ear. The patient had an enlarging tumor in the gland with suspicion of cancer. The difficulty with this surgery is that the facial nerve dives through it on its way to the facial muscles. To make matters worse, it sends off multiple tiny branches the size of thread. Since the facial nerve is responsible for facial movement, cutting the trunk would paralyze that half of the face. Cutting one of the smaller branches would paralyze part of the face. For instance, the patient would be able to do only a half-smile if the branch to the lips were damaged.

We made an incision just in front of the ear, snaking it around to the backside of the ear and then down the hairline, a "face-lift" incision that leaves a nearly-invisible scar. To my surprise, I was allowed to participate to a small degree, a pleasant surprise considering the fact that getting face-time with attending surgeons can be difficult. I attribute it to my eagerness before the surgery. Just by chance, I had walked out to scrub at the same time he did, striking up a conversation about my anticipation and interest in this particular procedure. He asked me detailed questions about the patient, testing me to see if I had read up on the case.

It would have been a disaster if I hadn't, because this guy was also the residency director. My answers must have been the right ones; I was rewarded by being able to perform a small amount of cutting with the harmonic, an instrument that clamps onto the highly vascularized gland and then burns its way through. This prevents excessive bleeding from obscuring our view of the facial nerve.

At the end of the surgery, the attending personally guided me through suturing part of the incision; unfortunately, the entire team was present, watching me fumble my way through. Before long we broke out the staple gun and finished the job that way. The experience was gratifying; I can definitely see myself doing parotids in my practice.

Another interesting case worth mentioning here was a choanal atresia. Basically, the back of a young boy's nose was closed off on one side with bone and tissue, a birth defect that can be quite dangerous if it blocks both sides. Since the surgery's highly complicated details prevent a complete explanation here, the surgical procedure can be summarized as using scopes and three flaps from inside the nose to re-create the nasal airway after the bone was drilled through. The flaps were so complicated I barely understood what they were doing during the surgery.

My second week began with a little scare in the OR quite similar to an episode back on my surgery rotation. We were performing a simple tube placement in the ears of a five-month-old when the breathing tube down his throat must have slipped out. The irritation caused the vocal cords to slam shut, something we call laryngospasm. All of a sudden monitors everywhere started beeping.

Let me describe the worst feeling in the world: watching an infant's heart rate drop from the 100s to the 90s, to the 80s, to the 70s, to the 60s, to the 50s. "Apnea" was flashing on the anesthesiologist's monitor, indicating no breaths were being taken. "Let's bag him!" the ENT resident said. They quickly pulled the breathing tube and began manual breaths for the child. For a while nothing seemed to help. The OR tech ran to the side of the room to kick the code blue button; just seconds before she did, the anesthesiology resident announced that he was coming out of it. While he demanded that everyone calm down, the technician still paged for any available anesthesiology attendings to come to the room.

Within seconds an attending burst through the doors asking questions and expecting quick answers. Technicians shortly followed asking if we needed the crash cart. By this time the vitals were beginning to normalize. However, the vitals took one more gigantic dip before finally stabilizing enough to reintubate him. A paralyzing agent was given to relax the vocal cords and open the airway. Chills rushed down my spine as I considered that a disaster had been avoided through the quick actions of the medical team. Afterwards, I asked the ENT resident how he knew what to do. He was only two short years ahead of me and looked like a pro. I hoped to be ready.

I can't imagine what it would have been like if we had lost that baby. In reality it wasn't that close of a call considering a paralytic agent usually does the trick. Still, I hoped never to see a patient die on the operating table, though it is a risk that exists in the life of every surgeon.

While the risks and benefits are explained thoroughly to every patient willing to go under the knife, allergic reactions to anesthesia drugs, losing the airway, and bleeding are a few side effects from any surgery that can cause death. The vast majority of the time nothing happens, and surgery is a wonderful thing. Still, I fear the rare complications.

The next case involving a young child was less thrilling but just as poignant. A 5-year-old suffered a severe case of respiratory papillomas, warty growths caused by the HPV virus. The HPV virus is often sexually transmitted, often resulting in genital warts and cervical cancer. The cause of respiratory papillomatosis is theorized to be infection during vaginal delivery. While surgery is used to eliminate them, they reoccur so often that the patient needs dozens of surgeries. Everyone in the room had to wear specialized masks to prevent airborne HPV from infecting our upper airways.

To look down the patient's throat, we used what amounted to a hollowed rod with a built-in light, vaporizing the papillomas with a laser. This procedure translates into a very tricky situation: a tube of highly flammable oxygen is only millimeters away from a hot laser. Considering this an important piece of information, the attending asked me what I would do if the airway caught on fire.

In an effort to save me, the resident behind him pantomimed the answer to me. "Yank out the breathing tube to cut off the oxygen supply," I answered correctly. When he asked what needed to be done before that, I had no answer.

The right answer turned out to be a frightening one: turn off the oxygen first and then pull the tube. Otherwise the tube would become a makeshift flame-thrower. It turns out he had seen an airway catch on fire during residency. However, everyone had moved so quickly in cutting off the fuel and pulling the tube that the patient did just fine. In addition to cutting off the fuel supply, the tube is pulled to collapse the tissues and smother the fire. I tucked away these bits of knowledge in case I am ever confronted with this in the future.

During this week, interview offers for residency began trickling in. By the end of the week, I had five scheduled throughout the Midwest, which relieved much of my fear of not matching in one of the most competitive fields in medicine. I had read that even high scores don't guarantee someone a spot in ENT. Getting an interview at the Mayo Clinic also helped to boost my confidence.

Still, while my confidence rose, so did financial obligations: no extra loan money is allotted for the extra expenses during fourth year, so I had to book the interviews and hotels straight to my credit card. The tabulations kept piling on. Adding this to the two-thousand needed for Step 2 of the boards, I was in quite a lot of credit card debt, in addition to my greater than $200,000 in loans. I tried to convince myself that it was just a number and in a few years I would have a great job and money coming in. Having a young wife and wanting to support her and a new family creates a pretty intimidating situation.

After a lot of soul searching, I resolved to just have fun with the interviews. Would I stay in Chicago as originally planned or would I allow myself to be lured away by another program? Should I take my wife to a new location where she doesn't know anyone while I work eighty hours a week? All of these questions were constantly on my mind as I tried to concentrate on my rotations.

I had to try and suppress some of this debate while I focused on my two remaining weeks of my audition rotation. The green service was much more laid back then the previous two weeks on the red team. Most of the surgeries involved the smaller, outpatient type procedures that ENT is known for. I saw a lot of pediatric ear tubes, tonsils, adenoids, and nasal surgery, certainly not as glamorous and exciting as the cancer surgeries, but cases I will see often in my own practice.

The reader shouldn't get the impression that we saw very little excitement. We had a thyroid case on an elderly woman, but it wasn't the surgery that interested me. This sweet old lady was actually a prisoner who was kept shackled by armed guards. Before she woke up from anesthesia following the surgery, we were left speechless after learning her background information. She had been a caretaker of a young, paralyzed patient whom she decided one day to beat to death. The entire room buzzed about the perverse details, all of us wondering how such a sweet lady could have such a dark side.

The following morning I arrived before the residents so I peeked in to see how she was doing. We had left a drain in her neck incision so I decided to check on it to make sure it wasn't clogged. A guard was still in the room by her bedside, guarding whom I have to admit was indeed the sweetest-acting grandma I had ever seen. Later, when the residents arrived, they instructed me to pull the drain from her neck since there was little output. She acted surprised when I told her she would be discharged that day, even asking when she would have to come back to clinic for her follow-up appointment. I recognized this as a desperate attempt to get away from prison for any period of time. Could there be any room for pity for a patient such as this? That's when I decided to push my thoughts and emotions to the back of my mind and remember the Hippocratic Oath. I am not to serve as judge and jury but to heal the sick, a promise for which I strive to maintain.

I shrugged the emotions off for my final week at UIC. I needed to focus and impress the residents and attendings so they would remember me as one of the good medical students. At this point, I had been in the OR for the majority of the previous six months. It had just started to become normal, almost mundane. That didn't last long.

Later that day we had finished cutting a deeply imbedded tumor out of a guy's neck, sacrificing the jugular vein in the process. Luckily, having another jugular on the other side of the neck usually suffices. All that was left to do was to place a drain in the neck and close up. The attending left the room to go talk to the pathologists while the resident, three years ahead of me in the learning curve, and I finished. After I made a small cut in the skin with a scalpel, he poked the drain through the skin and muscle into the newly created hole in the neck. A few moments later we noticed the neck wound was full of blood. "Was it dry before?" he asked. I replied that we had good hemostasis, or bleeding control, when the boss left.

We quickly suctioned it out to try and find the source, but as quickly as we suctioned, blood would reappear and obscure our view. "I bet I hit the EJ," he said, referring to the external jugular vein. The once lively OR had become quiet as everyone tried to listen to our conversation. Here we had a delay in the case, as well as the anticipation of a thoroughly pissed-off attending upon her return. Finally, we packed the wound to try to control the bleeding and simply waited for her. When she did return, she let us know of her anger in no uncertain terms.

After she scrubbed back in, she surprised us by asking questions about what had happened as if nothing was wrong. After the resident's delayed responses, she stated, "We're moving on," her way of letting him know that he should forget his mistake and just concentrate on fixing it.

All surgeons make mistakes; some can be helped and others can't. What I took out of that situation was to not to dwell on my mistakes with a patient on the table but instead to act quickly to correct problems. The important thing was to recognize that things can go awry, but they do not have to escalate into an unfixable situation.

Later in the week I had an interesting opportunity come my way. UIC's ENT program is well known for its specialty in facial plastic surgery. A couple of the higher-ups on staff are Otolaryngologists who fellowship-trained in facial plastics. I left UIC one day to scrub in with one of the surgeons at a surgicenter in downtown Chicago, a posh center right on Michigan Avenue. In the operating room on the fifteenth floor, I had a nice view of the Chicago skyline. The surgeon himself was one of the most famous rhinoplasty surgeons in the world. Every time I saw him he was decked out in a nice black suit, prompting me to wonder if someday I would dress that classy.

The surgery patient was a young guy whose nose was severely crooked from a prior tumor resection. He could hardly breathe through his nose so the surgery was mostly functional in nature, with cosmetics thrown in as a bonus. I learned that many of the rhinoplasty cases are similar to this. I'm sure most people think of plastic surgery as the appearance-only driven profession portrayed on television. In reality, many of their operations are functional or reconstructive in nature and very rewarding. Pictures of the nose from every possible angle were hung up on the wall for the surgeon to reference during surgery. The angle was right in line with the beautiful skyline, which gave me the perfect excuse to glance at the city in the early morning hours. I had been in Chicago for four years, but the skyline never got old.

We made an incision on the bottom of the nose and pulled the skin up towards the forehead completely exposing the cartilage and bone. Over the next five hours the nose was completely deconstructed and built back up again using cartilage harvested from both the nose and a rib. The other participants were a facial plastic surgery fellow and a visiting ENT resident from California, coming in to witness and learn this doctor's coveted technique. The most meticulous surgeon I had ever seen, he carved up the rib cartilage into rectangles, squares, and other shapes as needed. We stopped the surgery more than a dozen times to take pictures and check the alignment.

When we were done, a patchwork of tiny pieces of cartilage was sewn together, reconstituting a straight nose for the patient for the first time in his young life and allowing him to breathe more easily. I had a great time learning the difficult anatomy and surgical steps throughout the morning from this man. The atmosphere in the OR was very relaxed as we talked and laughed, a rarity in the OR as many surgeons are very intense. The surgicenter was called "900 North" since that was the address on Michigan Avenue.

At one point the fellow made a joke about getting his own reality TV show. I exclaimed that "900 North" sounded like a great name for a reality show, but they would likely have to wear sleeveless scrub shirts if they wanted to make it on MTV.

Ending the rotation by witnessing a new and difficult surgery for the first time was exhilarating. I will have to learn how to do rhinoplasties to fix broken and deviated noses. Whether or not I will do purely cosmetic facial plastic surgery will in part depend on how much exposure I get in my residency and also my interest in performing those surgeries.

The following day we did another rhinoplasty at UIC. The chief resident struggled through the case and exclaimed that many feel that it is the most difficult surgery in facial plastics and ENT. Whether or not this is true, I'm not certain, but it was an interesting operation. My last day was one of those "no breaks, no eating" days, so I was tired before the end. As this was my last surgical rotation of medical school, my adventures in the operating room were over for a long time.

129

Chapter 14: The Unit

Running the gauntlet is an ancient practice where warriors proved themselves to be adequate for battle through physical punishment. Many have no idea that this practice still exists in our society. It's called the surgical intensive care unit, where young doctors prove themselves to their superiors through painful hours and hard-core medicine. I am not saying this is a bad thing. I knew going into it that this month would be difficult but that I would come out of it feeling much closer to being a physician than ever before. Considering graduation was only nine months away, I was very hopeful this would be the case.

After orientation on our first day, the five "sub-Is", or fourth-year medical students training to be interns, gathered to make our schedule. Scheduling under our own judgment, one or two students had to be there at all hours of the day, night, weekday, and weekend. I began the month with a week of nights. I showed up each day around 5:30 PM and left around 8:00 AM the next day. The nights were fifteen-hours-long, depending on what was going on. We got one day off a week so that we didn't break the eighty-hour work-week limit.

I was so flustered on my first night I began to doubt my competency as a physician. The intensive care unit is where the sickest and most complicated patients in the hospital are housed. The sheer complexity of caring for them still boggles my mind. Everything from ventilator settings to procedures had to be learned in a short amount of time. I couldn't really fall back on my training in third-year since procedures and ICU material aren't the focus. Generally, we as students picked a couple of patients and concentrated on them for learning purposes.

On nights, however, the two of us had to be responsible for entire pods, or sections, of the ICU with about ten patients each. I performed miserably the first night, never knowing what was going on with my patients and having to fall back on the resident. He was a second-year, general-surgery resident and responsible for the care of all twenty-five to thirty-five patients in the entire ICU. A senior resident supervised him, but, mainly, he napped in the residents' room until something came up. The hierarchy in medicine is beautifully illustrated here.

The trauma surgeons run the SICU since the vast majority of patients are traumas. This meant that my team would run the traumas and even do the operating, if needed. However, since the month was geared toward learning to be an intern, I missed out on a lot of the excitement. When work needed to be done in the unit, I stayed behind to get it done. In fact, on my second night, I missed out on an exploratory laparotomy for a gunshot wound to the abdomen. When I heard the "TRAUMA CODE RED" over the speakers in the hospital, you would have thought I was missing out on my own graduation party. Being scrubbed into a life-and-death operation is an adrenaline rush like no other.

That patient was not the last one to come to us that night for gunshot wounds. Apparently, a gunman had walked into a crowded area and begun spraying bullets, making me really proud to live in Chicago. It wasn't long before I heard "PEDIATRIC TRAUMA CODE RED" over the speakers. I did make it to this one.

It was a young, teenage boy who had received some buckshot in his abdomen. He wasn't serious enough to go to the OR; so, after examining him, I left to get more work done in the unit. I know that at least one person died from that incident because I read about it in the news when I got home. In fact, I made it a habit after each shift to check the news for information about the patients I had just treated.

From motor vehicle accidents to attempted homicides, I saw it all that month. On my first night I took care of patients ranging from a patient fresh out of a kidney transplant to a woman hit by a train. The unfortunate woman had tried to beat a train but didn't make it; her kids were dead at the scene. She had so many broken bones and injuries I am surprised she made it as long as she did. The neurosurgeons bolted her head in place because any small movement of her broken neck could have killed her. A nurse once asked the resident what her "atlanto-occipital fracture" was. He replied, "It basically means that her head isn't attached to her neck." She died a few days later after the family decided to pull the plug.

One of the most common procedures performed in an ICU is an arterial line placement. This simply involves sticking a line in the radial artery of the wrist for blood draws. Arterial blood is more important to measure in sick patients than venous blood because it gives us an idea of how well the blood is being oxygenated. I assisted the resident on a difficult patient. She was ventilated but conscious enough to writhe in pain each time she was stuck. The main problem was that she moved every time he got the placement. Consequently, we spent over an hour digging a sharp needle into her arm before we were successful.

Shortly thereafter another patient lost her a-line. Frustrated by the time wasted on the first patient, the resident sent me to do my first a-line alone. I awkwardly gathered my supplies with the help of the nurse. I pretended to know what I was doing, ashamed of the lack of experience but delighted to get the first one over with. Quite a few minutes were spent feeling for the radial pulse, half of which was actually going over the procedure in my head. Unfortunately for both of us, she had terrible swelling which made her pulse difficult to feel.

After cleaning the area with alcohol, I took out the needle and pierced her skin at a 45-degree angle. The skin was surprisingly difficult to break. I went directly for the area where I had felt the pulse, to no avail. After backing the needle up, I angled it differently before plunging the needle in again. I tried over and over again, each time going deeper with the needle. I soon realized this wasn't going to be an easy stick. A stronger pulse could be palpated on the other wrist so I moved over to it for a try.

By this time I was getting exhausted and careless. After pulling the needle out, I slipped and plunged the dirty needle right into my finger. There was hardly any pain so I didn't know for sure if I was punctured until I pulled off my glove to see the blood.

Getting a needle stick isn't nearly as scary the second time around. The patient seemed like a harmless old lady to me, but one can never be certain. I followed the protocols and went home for the day since the morning had come. This left me only five hours to sleep before heading back in. When I arrived the following evening, this patient still had no arterial access. The residents couldn't get it either and apparently abandoned the task for more important things. Both of her wrists had dozens of tiny puncture attempts. Later in the night a resident and I tried again, only this time we went for the large artery in the groin that feeds the leg.

My job was to hold the "pannus," or fat rolls, back while the resident bored a four-inch long needle deep into her groin. Sadly, the central line was just as difficult. He jabbed the needle in and out in sort of a search-and-destroy technique. I don't even want to guess at how many times he attempted the puncture. Thankfully, she was almost completely sedated to make her comfortable on the ventilator and likely felt very little of the pain. The resident finally gave up and left the room. On his way out he told me to try the radial again. I looked at the dozens of failed attempts on her wrists and had little confidence in myself that I could succeed.

This time I was bolder in my attempts. I got an arterial Doppler and mapped out the artery using sound waves. I also went deeper, thinking that I might be missing the artery due to the swelling and edema. Sometimes you can feel the artery as you are piercing it. As you are moving the needle, it is soft in the fat until you meet the resistance of the muscular arterial wall. I thought I'd found this resistance at one point; but, after giving a little more force, I realized it was bone.

I cringed at that moment as I still cringe now when thinking about it. It must have been painful, fentanyl or not. I quickly backed it out and focused my probing a little more superficially. All of a sudden, there it was. The flash of blood indicating my needle was in the artery. My left hand slid the guide wire down as my right hand steadied the needle. At this point, I froze: I couldn't remember for the life of me what the next step was. My heart started racing as I focused as hard as I could on the night before when I watched the resident put in a line.

The pressure mounted as I had already proclaimed my success to the nurse in the room. His full attention was on my amazing success as I stood there like an idiot. Finally, I asked him to get the resident. The junior resident had stepped out so only the chief was available. By the time he walked in, I had lost the artery. Talk about an embarrassing moment. You can bet I never forgot the steps of an a-line after that. It is very simple, but I simply froze from inexperience.

By the third night I was feeling much more comfortable in my new role. The resident must have noticed this and took full advantage of it. Each time a new patient was added to the service, a lot of work was involved. Five patients were added that night, and I did the consult notes on all of them. It was a great learning experience but a lot of work, since I still moved slowly. A resident could do it rather quickly, but the complexity of the patients had me moving at a turtle's pace.

As I finished my fifth note, I heard that a serious trauma was on the way.

I rushed to the trauma bay to find the residents and trauma surgeon already at work. An elderly man lay on the table surrounded by people. The first thing I noticed was his bloody head, the second was the heart monitor showing ventricular fibrillation. "You're going to see someone die," I thought to myself.

I got from the nurses that he was a fall victim but no other information was known at the time. A couple of Emergency Medicine docs also came in to assist with the resuscitation. We shocked him twice and got his heart back into a sinus rhythm.

After he was examined and stabilized, we rushed him into the CT scanner. The first priority was imaging his head. We transported him onto the scanner, being careful to stabilize his spine. From around the pool of blood forming on the ground below, I carefully walked into the control room. We all huddled around the CT technician to see the images in real time. The scan showed massive intra-cranial bleeding as well as fractures of the skull base.

It takes a pretty strong impact to cause such devastation. The fracture also went through the orbit, which explained the large swelling in his right eye. The patient was deemed inoperable and the decision made to tell the family. He was taken to the unit briefly to give the family time to absorb the situation before withdrawing support.

It's interesting how different two nights can be in the hospital. One night I did consult notes for the resident the entire night, which is boring and labor-intensive.

The following night was completely hands-on and interactive. The first trauma code red of the night was a motorcycle crash victim. As I walked into the trauma bay, an entire team of people was waiting already, with what had to have been fifteen in the crowded room. The scene was reminiscent of the doctors on the television show *ER* waiting in great expectation for the incoming trauma. The trauma surgeon must have deemed the buzz a little too much and began throwing people out who didn't belong.

When the paramedics wheeled the patient in, all I could see was a blood-covered face. Apparently he had collided headfirst into a pole, and the pole had won. He was a burly man, with large tattoos over his torso and a rough demeanor. I sighed when I heard he had not been wearing a helmet. I knew the injuries would now be much greater than they had to be.

We suctioned the oozing blood from his mouth and nostrils so it wouldn't occlude the airway. An anesthesiology resident intubated him so we wouldn't lose his airway. After the primary and secondary surveys were over, we performed a chest x-ray and took him to CT. The imaging showed massive facial bone fractures going all the way back to the base of the skull. His forehead bone was also broken, leaving a soft spot covered by skin lacerations. I put a catheter into his penis since he wouldn't be going to the bathroom on his own for awhile.

Getting a procedure in a hard-core trauma is a major plus for a medical student, and I guess I must have impressed the chief. My hands flew faster than ever before as I inserted the catheter via sterile technique. If I was too slow, I would have quickly been replaced with a resident. After most of the work was done, I had a few seconds to look around at the scene before me. The floor was covered in bloody footprints tracked back and forth across the room. I remember this image quite distinctly; this was the moment of decision when I began storing my shoes in a plastic bag when I got home each night.

Upon this patient's arrival in the SICU, multiple teams were fighting for their time. The neurosurgeons were there to evaluate his neurological status. I was there fighting to put in an arterial line. The nurses were there to take vitals and labs. The facial plastics guy was there to sew up the lacerations on his face. The neurosurgeons determined that he didn't need his head bolted into place. With that taken care of, I jumped in to place an arterial line.

Since he constantly jerked his arm away in spite of the restraints, I found it to be another difficult stick. At one point he jerked his arm, and I felt bone again. Apparently I hadn't learned my lesson from the previous incident. I chastised myself but quickly moved on to focus on the procedure even though it angered me that the five or more people in the room wouldn't at least pin his arm down. I began to wonder if I was being hazed.

By this point the resident grew impatient and began trying an a-line on the other wrist. She had little success as well, so I didn't feel as embarrassed in front of everyone. A neurosurgery resident eventually placed the line. The last guy to get his turn on the patient was the resident on facial plastic surgery call. He was an intern in orthopedics rotating through plastics. He was also a Loyola graduate in the class before mine. It was interesting to see a glimpse of the responsibilities I would have in exactly one year, since ENT residents also take facial trauma call.

I stayed around to help him since I was interested in facial trauma repair. As we sewed up the guy's face, he writhed and tried to scream. He could not, however, due to the breathing tube down his throat and the restraints holding down his arms, not to mention the fact that his eyes were nearly swollen shut. I felt bad for the guy; he must have felt trapped and miserable. Imagine not being able to communicate, all the while being stuck with painful needles. Being a trauma patient is one thing I would like to avoid in this life.

At one point the resident left to answer a page. We had the patient's face covered in sterile draping, and he couldn't see anything. All of a sudden, he began shaking violently. I tried to ask what he needed, but I couldn't understand his moans. I didn't have to wait long for my answer as a gush of blood began pouring out of his mouth. My hand reached for the suction to clean out his mouth. Blood must have drained down from his sinuses and collected in the back of his throat.

I stared at the rainbow of tattoos on his body as the intern sewed up his face. While he sutured the laceration on his forehead, the skin depressed like jelly with pressure from the needle. The frontal bones had been crushed in the impact. This worried me because I didn't want the needle to get the brain, yet I kept my mouth shut since saying anything like that would have nearly scared the patient to death. Besides, the intern knew what he was doing.

I had spent a lot of time away from my work in the SICU and knew that work was backing up. The resident, a fellow classmate, and I split up the three pods in the ICU to begin updating the computers and checking on labs and x-rays. My work wasn't nearly completed before another trauma came in. The resident sent me down to see if the chief and intern needed help. The patient had gotten drunk at a wedding and fallen down a flight of stairs. He had already been evaluated at an outside hospital and had been found to have a wrist fracture and a small contusion on the brain.

It was going to be a fairly straightforward code. To my delight, the chief sat this one out so I could run the code with only the intern. My excitement built as we waited for the patient to arrive. He went over the trauma algorithm and described what I should do.

When the patient finally arrived, we transported him onto the bed. He was surprisingly bloody for a fall patient. His wrist was swollen and deformed from the fracture. After we asked him his name, we knew his airway was intact since he spoke.

Next, we checked for breathing with our stethoscopes and shouted "lungs clear to auscultation" to the nurse recording everything. Circulation was next, and I palpated the arteries and shouted, "Fems palpable bilaterally. DPs palpable bilaterally." After rolling him onto his side, I checked for spine fractures by rolling my fingers from the base of his skull all the way down his back, feeling for step-offs and trying to induce pain.

When I reached his buttocks, I lubricated my gloved finger and inserted it into his rectum. "There is positive rectal tone and stool in the vault," I said to the nurse. "No gross blood." There were many other steps of the exam as the entire body is inspected for injury. My first trauma code was a success, and my confidence began to build.

Many other interesting patients arrived in my first week of nights. We admitted one suicide attempt who had stabbed himself six or seven times in the chest and neck. His heart had even been pierced, but somehow he survived. Another guy had been beaten in the head with a baseball bat until his bones were crushed. A hunter paralyzed after falling out of a tree became the fourteenth person in the world to grow a rare species of bacteria. And, last but not least, I saw multiple motor vehicle crash patients. Enough pain and misery passed through in one night in the unit to last a lifetime.

While the key is to separate the emotion from the care just enough to function properly, it's important not to become completely ambivalent.

Switching to days was much easier than switching to nights. Although I was still working fourteen to fifteen hour days, six days a week, it didn't seem as bad when sleeping next to my wife every night. The day shifts had much more formality to deal with. The mornings consisted of radiology rounds with the attending followed by patient rounds. The trauma service is so large that rounding took all morning. We all showed up around 5 AM to pre-round on all of the patients. The medical students then had the unfortunate task of printing and photocopying every note for everyone on the team, an ugly secretarial task that we despised.

To make matters worse, the trauma attendings can be a bit demanding at times. The residents were verbally pummeled on rounds for not knowing the answers to something asked. If a complication arose on their watch, rounding would be miserable. I took it in stride like everything else so it wasn't too bad. Dwelling on the situation only makes it worse psychologically, especially when one is exhausted.

During the afternoon and early evening, my job was very similar to the night shift. Writing consult notes on new patients, helping run traumas, and updating the computer logs on patients were some of my responsibilities. The first trauma I went to during the day was a facial trauma.

Because they all knew of my interest in ENT, the residents always got excited for me anytime we received word of facial trauma: "Hey, Brandon, we've got the perfect trauma coming in for you. Some guy's nose fell off," a resident once said. Apparently, some guy who hadn't been wearing a seat belt had crashed into a stopped car.

When the paramedics brought him in, they said his face had gone through the windshield and then back again into the car. His entire face was covered in blood because of extreme lacerations, the worst being at the nose. The left half of his nose was nearly cut off.

Some gauze had been stuffed under it to coagulate the bleeding. This, however, only made the appearance more frightening as the nose stuck out into the air in an abnormal fashion. The oral surgery team was consulted as they split the facial trauma call with plastics and ENT. Today was their day to shine.

I began to get a little braver during trauma codes. When it was time to roll the patient over to check for injuries on his back, I went to the head of the patient to secure his neck. He had a neck collar on, but someone still needed to brace it for protection. I placed my hands on his head the best I could. I was staring straight down into his deformed face while he moaned in agony. "You're holding it wrong!" the resident shouted as he showed me the proper way to brace it.

Holding his head in place while we rolled him on his side was surprisingly difficult. The intern took almost a minute to check his back for step-offs and to perform a rectal exam. We sent the guy to the scanner and let oral surgery button him up.

He was very fortunate that he didn't have any more serious injuries. He had some fractures to his nasal bones, but that was it. I wrote the transfer note a few days later when he was leaving our unit. I took one last peek at his face, and it looked quite nice. It still would have gagged most people outside of the medical field, but, comparatively speaking, he looked great.

The following morning was dobhoff day. The dobhoff is a tube snaked through a patient's nose down to his or her stomach for the purpose of feeding. I mentioned that I hadn't had the chance to do one and my fellow sub-Is and residents acted surprised.

By lunch I had performed at least three and one or two the following day. One patient in particular was not being very cooperative. She kept pulling out her dobhoff and having to get it replaced. This happened three or four times. She spoke only Spanish, so I had my classmate come and scold her every time, explaining why she needed it.

Patients get a little bit disoriented in the unit so I never took it personally. The key to placing the tube is to go straight back and not angle it upward, following the external contour of the nose. Because this usually gags the patient a little, it's important to move quickly. Only once did it come out of the patient's mouth; unfortunately, my resident had to be watching that time.

To make sure the tube is in the stomach you simply place your stethoscope over the abdomen and listen as you blow air into the tube with a syringe. The noise is unmistakable.

Although placing dobhoff tubes is about as simple of a procedure there is, it felt good to have one more notch on my belt. After that point whenever a resident needed help with dobhoffs I could offer without having to be taught how. As an intern, I will be expected to do all of this anyway so any experience is good experience.

As I was about to leave to end my second week on the rotation, another trauma was announced over the loud speakers. I debated at first whether to go since the night team was on their way in. Heading to a trauma that late could add hours onto my already-long fourteen-hour day. I followed my gut instincts and ran down to the bay.

I arrived before the patient for once and asked what the situation was. A young guy, about my age, had fallen down an elevator shaft, landing on debris below which made jagged cuts into his body. He was flown in via helicopter and was not in good shape.

While he moaned in agony, we tried unsuccessfully to get good information from him: he spoke only Russian and was unable to communicate. He did speak the universal language of pain, however, which allowed us to elucidate where the main problems were. We began our examination in earnest and quickly found that he had no sensation or motor movement in his legs. He was paralyzed at the age of twenty-three.

We rolled him over as usual and found some impressive lacerations. Huge flaps of bloody tissue could be seen across his back. It was apparent that he landed on his back. The chief told me to put a Foley catheter into his bladder. Since I had performed dozens of these, I didn't think much about it, but a problem developed because I had been sweating from all of the action. When I tried to put on the sterile gloves, they wouldn't go on. The chief became more and more impatient as I struggled. I finally had to try inserting the Foley with the sterile gloves only halfway on.

"Have you done this before?" the chief asked. "Yes," was my obvious answer since he had already watched me put one in. "Well, then get to it!" I put the Foley in but not before he found one or two more things I was doing wrong. The junior resident also snapped at me during the trauma for not having scissors ready to cut off the clothes.

It was a stressful time, but I let the comments slide off me. When we took the patient to the scanner, I could hear him moaning in agony. The technicians kept trying to still him so his movements wouldn't mess up the images. They took breaks while the nurse would run in to snow him with more sedative.

While we were standing there, we heard the announcement of a pediatric trauma. I ran back into the trauma bay right behind the residents; and, in our hurry into the bay, we apparently and inadvertently cut off some ER technician who was wheeling a patient into one of the rooms. "I was just taking him right here so you could have waited!" she snarled. "Ignorant!" None of us even looked back because we had a child to save, a thirteen-year-old girl who had been run over by a car.

When they brought her in, she was crying from the pain. A tire-track mark snaked up her body and over half her face. The most fascinating part about the scenario was not the trauma but the fact that she begged us not to cut off her jeans. The girl was concerned about her pants even when her life could have been in jeopardy.

We cut them off anyway because sliding off jeans takes too long and could injure her even worse. I held her head when we rolled her, trying to comfort her during the uncomfortable and painful process of having her body propped sideways. After imaging her, we found fractured bones and some small injuries to her abdominal organs but nothing life threatening. I was thankful for this.

Seeing a young girl hurt like that was difficult, and, leaving that day, I had a weird feeling. It felt good to be part of saving a girl's life, but at the same time, I was reeling from the chaos and the multiple scoldings. I used it to toughen myself. Rarely do I tell my wife about the terrible things I see at work. I don't like to bother her with the burdens I choose to carry. That night was different though. I needed someone to talk with and she, of course, was there for me.

The next week or so was nothing special. I cut back my trauma time for the more mundane ICU work, a necessary evil because I needed to be able to manage the sickest patients in the hospital as an intern. Every now and then the residents would teach me a new procedure. Each day I felt more and more comfortable in the ICU. What was once intimidating was becoming more manageable.

The traumas seemed to come in phases. We may have gone days without penetrating trauma to then get a slew of them all at once. One day was 'Gunshot Wound Day', while the next was 'Dropped Baby Day'. "Dropping baby" is more like "shake and throw baby" half the time. A serious skull fracture requires an acute force. Simply claiming he or she fell off the couch doesn't cut it in the trauma bay. An investigation usually ensues.

I went to one of the baby traumas. She looked so tiny on the board on which they wheeled her in that my heart dropped. I have a serious soft spot for kids. She had a small amount of bleeding on the brain but was otherwise okay. She was about five-months-old and screamed the entire time we examined her. Afterwards I spent about ten minutes just playing with her. I had her calmed down and sucking on her pacifier in no time. Another child wasn't so lucky: a major skull fracture was discovered.

The trauma service can identify the day when the Chicago PD decides to bust the drug dealers. That was 'Gunshot Wound Day'. The first patient had been shot through the head and was pronounced dead in the trauma bay. I looked up his head scan out of curiosity and could see the bullet's trajectory quite well. The second patient had tried to run from the cops, which was his first mistake. His second was trying to run over a few of them in his car. They shot him multiple times. He was taken for emergency surgery to save his life.

It was a pack and "Get the heck out of Dodge" kind of case. The only objective was to eliminate life threatening injuries such as hemorrhage and then to get out before he died on the table. The trauma surgeon left the abdominal incision open but very well bandaged. After the damage control and a couple of days to stabilize, he was taken back to the OR for a complete tuning up.

Meanwhile, the police shackled his feet to the bed and camped outside his room the entire time. Some of the residents made a fuss over it, but I say let them do their job. Patients have escaped from hospitals before with terrible injuries. However, I'm guessing we stopped any escape plans he may have had when we told him his abdomen was splayed open.

The third gunshot victim that day had been driving with his girlfriend when a car crashed into them. A jealous ex-boyfriend then got out of the car and began spraying them with bullets. The guy took one to the chest and was brought to Loyola. He was bleeding internally so the decision was made to place a chest tube. Even though a little numbing medicine was injected into his side, it never quite does the job. Getting a chest tube is a very painful experience. Patients usually scream the entire time. The tubing is then connected to a vacuum that sucks out the blood inside the chest. This guy was quite lucky considering the high-priced real estate in the bullet's trajectory. Bone fragments were millimeters away from the largest artery in the body, the aorta. He was able to be managed non-operatively and was spared a sternotomy.

I actually got to pull a chest tube on one of our patients. A huge bandage about two-feet in length is made of paper tape. Some gauze soaked in Vaseline is layered on top to seal off the open wound. If any air gets into the wound while pulling the tube, the lung could collapse. The lungs are held open with a vacuum-like pressure in the chest. If the chest tube is not pulled fast enough, or if the bandage is not airtight, the lung can collapse causing respiratory distress. I had an intern helping me so it wasn't that big of a deal.

One other procedure I learned was changing a central line over a wire. Granted, it's not as interesting as placing the central line in the first place, but I can live with that. A central line is simply a large IV placed into one of the major veins in the body. These procedures are major for us as students because of the complications associated with them. If you miss the jugular in the neck, you can hit the carotid artery, which is under extremely high pressure. Blood could literally arc across the room. Missing the subclavian vein below the clavicle could cause a pneumothorax, or collapsed lung. A chest tube would then have to be placed.

Consequently, medical students aren't first on the list to put in central lines. We can, however, change them over a wire. It is still quite complicated at first. The patient's bed is adjusted so the feet are up in the air in order to prevent an air embolus from traveling to the brain and causing a stroke. If the air bubble rises, it will go to the heart and then the periphery of the body, where it will be absorbed. It is an extremely small risk, but precautions are taken nonetheless. The poor lady I performed my second one on was a post-operative patient with pain issues. She cried and moaned the entire time. It is very unnerving to cause so much pain. Most of it was due to her bad back, but I couldn't help but feel it was partly my fault. Adding to the pressure was the fact that it was only my second time doing this procedure. The resident expected me to know how to do it. Right off the bat I forgot two steps. The patient's threatening to rip off the draping didn't help the situation. That's when I decided that I like operating much more than doing procedures. I like my patients asleep and with adequate analgesia.

Because of the way the scheduling worked out, I had a stretch of about nine days in a row without a day off. The fourteen to fifteen hour days without a break can wear on a person quickly. My last day of that particular week was a Saturday. I hoped the residents would let me off early since our final was the following week. That day turned out to be one of the most interesting of medical school. Every now and then someone will ask me if medical school is like the television show *ER*. I usually laugh because I think my life is mostly mundane. Yet that Saturday would be comparable to a season finale of *ER*. We began the day with our usual rounding on the ICU patients. Everything was going normally until we were halfway through the ICU. I should have known the day was jinxed when a code was called to the hospital cafeteria. The chief resident and my classmate had broken off to operate on the aforementioned gunshot victim. Right after they left, one of the junior residents was paged about a floor patient having a seizure. He had to run and check on the situation. Not even a minute had gone by before a trauma code red was announced.

I had my pick of a few interesting options, and I ended up choosing the trauma bay. This was the first day we didn't complete rounds, which was highly unusual. When they wheeled the woman in, she screamed in pain with every movement. She had fallen off a horse and was trampled in the process. We knew from the outside hospital from which she had been transferred that she had suffered multiple pelvic fractures. I now understood the screaming: if there is one thing I learned from this experience, it is that pelvic fractures are excruciating. The orthopedic surgeons were consulted, and we worked together to treat the patient.

The attending ordered CT scans to further evaluate her injuries. Before we sent her to the scans, the attending did a quick ultrasound of the abdomen. When she moved the probe to the right side of the abdomen she said, "Cancel the CT scans; we're going to the OR for emergency surgery." On the fuzzy ultrasound screen, I could see a small black space next to the liver; blood was accumulating in the gutters of the abdomen. The patient had internal bleeding. Her blood pressure began to drop as we rushed her to the OR. We split her abdomen open to explore the abdominal cavity. Meanwhile, the orthopedic surgeons were arriving to make plans for the pelvis. As we ran the bowel, we discovered multiple injuries. Luckily, none of them penetrated completely through the intestines spilling the stool, an injury capable of causing sepsis and death.

In the meantime, the chief resident had finished the gunshot case and began scrubbing into ours. He bumped out the junior resident according to the hierarchy. While they sewed many of the tears, the colon was beyond saving. More than half of it had to be removed. Cutting out bowel had to be done with the utmost care. They removed the damaged portion and hand-sutured the two ends together. A laceration to the liver was also found during the exploration. No resection was necessary.

As we scrubbed out, the orthopods took over. One of the residents noticed a small cut on the thigh. I later learned that the pelvis had fractured so badly that one of the bones had cut through the skin. This meant the bones were contaminated. What amounted to a clearing operation had to be performed in that area to stave off a raging bone infection. I wanted to stay to see them drill pins into her pelvis for stabilization, but there was too much work to do. She would have to go back for more orthopedic surgery a couple of days later when she was more stable.

Right as I left the OR, another trauma came in. A motorcyclist without a helmet was thrown thirty feet. Without a doubt we found skull fractures on his CT scan. While reading the scans, I took a ten-second lunch break and ate the granola bar I never had time to eat for breakfast. That's when things started to get really crazy.

A trauma code red was announced. I ran to the trauma bay in time to see another man brought in after crashing his motorcycle. He had not been wearing a helmet either and had suffered severe skull injuries. The injuries were so bad brain matter was coming out of his ears. As we palpated his body, we felt multiple bone fractures.

Neurosurgery was consulted, and they were having just as bad a day as we were. I heard one of the chief residents shouting on the phone that she hadn't been spread this thin in six years of residency. I thought it couldn't get any worse than this until one of the trauma nurses said that two more code reds were on the way. Before we let the brain surgeons take our patient to the OR, we needed to rule out internal bleeding. Shock from bleeding out is the most imminent threat to life in trauma patients. Due to his large belly, the FAST ultrasound was inadequate to rule out bleeding. The attending ordered a diagnostic peritoneal lavage.

A DPL tests for blood by jamming a large needle right into the belly. A wire is inserted through the needle. The needle is then pulled and a catheter is guided over the wire. A syringe is used to suck out any blood giving the diagnosis. If no blood is found, as in this case, a liter of saline is injected through the hole and sucked back out for testing. The patient was sent for surgery in the meantime. It was neurosurgery turf now so I stayed in the trauma bay. The patient's pupils were blown so his prognosis was extremely grave. A blown, or dilated pupil, means that the brain is herniating and compressing the nerve that constricts the pupil.

During all of the commotion, the CT scanner broke. Imagine the looks on our faces when we heard that news. To add insult to injury, the Intranet system that allows us to look up films was going off-line later in the evening for maintenance. Luckily, the problem with the CT scanner was quickly fixed and it was quickly put to good use.

The last trauma I helped with that day was a soccer player who got kicked in the head. She wasn't nearly as serious as the previous patient, so I got some practice with the FAST machine. It was a great way to learn considering the situation was more laid back and the chief wasn't in the room.

One more trauma code red was on the way when I left. I tried to stay, but the resident literally kicked me out. She was looking out for me and knew I was staying too late. That is the only problem with the eighty-hour-work-week limit. Sometimes you miss out on great learning opportunities. After I changed out of my scrubs and began walking out of the building, I heard the trauma announcement. Part of me wanted to go to it while part of me wanted to go home and eat my first meal of the day. I chose the latter. As I reflected on the events of the day, I was reminded of why I went into medicine. It took hours for the adrenaline rush to wind down.

During my last week in the unit I became much more worried about my upcoming exam than about going to all of the traumas. I had hoped they would let us off early to study but that didn't happen. The one thing that did happen was a surprising development of confidence in the last two days. The unit became much less intimidating and our role as students grew profoundly. Nurses began asking us questions about patients and, conversely, not asking us questions when we went to perform procedures on them. The nurses in the unit can be very protective of their patients and were the most difficult to win over.

The residents also had more confidence in our abilities and we proved to be a lot of help. After rounds, the work would be divided and we functioned just as residents. We couldn't put in orders for medications so, while the residents performed those functions, the procedures fell to us. I've already discussed the placement of a nasogastric tube down a patient's nose, but an event happened to me in the last week that would have been traumatizing had it not been so hilarious.

I was asked to place the NG tube in a young guy who had been shot in the abdomen. A huge gastric bubble was seen on X-ray that morning so we knew he was distended. The bowels often slow down after a traumatic event or surgery. He was restrained, as he was also under arrest, so the nurse decided to assist me. Looking back now I am thankful she decided to stick around. As I walked into the room, the guy was moaning in his bed and wouldn't respond to anything I said. I measured out the tubing and lubricated it to ease its passage to the stomach.

The moment the tubing hit his nose he began violently shaking his head. The nurse held him down, and I quickly passed the tubing down. Green gastric contents began coming up the tube almost as soon as it got into the stomach. I could tell immediately that the gastric contents were under pressure. The nurse knew what was coming and quickly connected the tube to the wall vacuum to suction it out. It was too late. All of a sudden, bright green vomit began spraying out of his mouth all of the way across the room. I placed my hand in front of the jet stream to prevent it from spraying on us as he violently shook his head. In seconds most of the bedding and floor below was drenched in vomit. I am talking *Exorcism* type of vomiting. In fact, I would almost swear that his head was spinning. The smell was nearly more than I could bear as a fourth-year medical student. That's when the guy really lost it and began shaking his head splattering me with vomit. Another nurse rushed in and put a mask on me while I bravely held the tubing in his nose so it wouldn't fall out.

I tried in vain to calm him down but nothing would work. He may have been in some sort of delirium.

After a few minutes, we had the stomach suctioned and the patient calmed down. The nurses gave me props for staying in the thick of it while being sprayed with vomit. The nurse was laughing out loud the entire time. Apparently, she had seen this type of stuff so many times it didn't faze her anymore. As I stepped back from it all, I noticed that the police officer that never leaves the room was nowhere to be seen. Apparently, the scene was a little too much even for him. I let the nurses clean up the mess since I wanted to wash my face in the break room. I inspected my white coat to find little green spots all over the sleeves. The worst part about the whole incident was that I was so overworked and exhausted I didn't wash my white coat for two days. I'm not proud of it, but that's what happens when you're working eighty hours a week.

After that incident I decided there was a little excitement yet to be had on this rotation so I went to the next two traumas. The first was a young boy involved in a car crash. He wasn't hurt badly, but the reason I mention him is that his dad ran from the scene and left him there alone. He must have been running from the cops, but I can't imagine how anyone could do such a thing. We shipped him off to the pediatric service to handle the social issues.

The next trauma was a code red. An elderly woman had jumped out of a third story window to commit suicide. She was transferred from an outside hospital so we knew she had pelvic and leg fractures. We rushed her to the operating room since her blood pressure was dropping.

As we wheeled her out of the trauma bay, the patient's daughter ran with us. At first, the rest of team didn't know she and the chaplain were right behind us. I prayed no one would say anything inappropriate about the patient's prognosis. When we stopped at the elevator, the daughter took the few moments afforded to her to talk to her mother. Tears began to fill her eyes, and she sobbed right there in the lobby over her broken mother. A family with two young children was also waiting for the elevator. I wondered what they had to be thinking. I found it difficult to hear her crying like that. I wanted to separate myself from the situation so I could focus on the case. "Separate yourself," I thought to myself as she cried and prayed in her Polish language.

In the OR we had to get better IV access before we could proceed. A simple IV line wouldn't cut it because massive transfusions were needed to keep her alive. The trauma fellow and chief resident worked on the right wrist. The anesthesiologist attending took the large vein in the neck. The anesthesiology resident took the left wrist. It was a beehive of activity as they all rushed to put in the lines. While Johnny Cash was blaring in the background, I couldn't help but get chills down my spine with the scene before me. Trauma surgery can be quite exhilarating.

When everything was ready, we cut into her belly but not into the peritoneum, the sack that contains the organs. The attending had me stick my hand down into the pelvis where I could feel the jagged, fractured bones. We packed her pelvis with sterile gauze and got out. The packing was used only to stop hemorrhaging and nothing else. She would have to return to the OR when she was more stable to get them removed. I later learned that the orthopods would not attempt to operate on her pelvis because it was fractured so badly that they were scared to get into it. The prognosis was bad and medical management would have to suffice. She would probably never walk again anyway.

The last exciting event in the SICU I witnessed was late at night as the day team was about to leave. The residents went to the conference room to sign out to the night team. I was the only medical personnel in the West Pod when a nurse yelled for help. I ran into the room to see an elderly patient slumped over her chair. Another medical student arrived at the same time. I yelled for her to find the residents. When she didn't move immediately, I ran to do it myself. I burst into the conference room and exclaimed, "We may have a code!" Now I expected everyone to rise in one accord and frantically run into the patient's room.

It was quite the opposite occurrence. They calmly asked me questions as they got up and walked with me to the room. I remember one of them being a little bit smart with me by saying, "What do you mean *you think* a patient is coding?" I quickly explained the nurse simply yelled for help, and I came to get them. In retrospect, I should have taken a few seconds to gather some information before bailing for help. In seconds the room was filled with people. We moved the patient into the bed and medication orders were yelled out.

The on-call anesthesiologists rushed in, panting from the long run from their call room. We intubated the patient and placed her on a ventilator to protect her airway. A nurse reported that she had been talking to a family member on the phone and complained of difficulty breathing before the phone went dead. The family was hysterical as you can imagine.

As we were busy working, her middle-aged son walked up to the door carrying his half-eaten dinner. The nurse quickly closed the curtain and went out to meet him. "She's having some problems," the nurse said. I'll never forget the look on his face when she said that. It was a look of terror in his eyes unlike anything I had ever seen. He was escorted to the visitor's room so we could finish our work. By the time we stabilized her, it was an hour over our shift's end, making it over a fifteen hour day. It was another one of those days when fatigue didn't touch me until I got home. The adrenaline was pumping, and I couldn't stop thinking about the event.

As I was leaving, the attending that operated on her that day showed up to see her with his residents trailing him. The vascular residents had been there within minutes and likely called him in from home. I found myself wondering about her that night. I couldn't wait to get there the next day to find out if she survived. I memorized everything the residents did so I would know what to do when it was my turn to make the decisions. The patient ended up being fine, and no cause was ever discovered.

My last day in the SICU capped it all off. New residents rotated onto the service, and we knew more about the unit than they did. It felt good to answer their questions and show off what we had learned that month. Even the nurses came to us with questions about what to do for their patients.

Although the rotation was tough, I learned a lot about managing the sickest patients in the hospital. I also realized, as usual, how much further I had to go to become the doctor I dreamed of becoming.

We also picked up some of the resident-level work, such as calling other services and consulting them to see patients. Not that it is rocket science, but communicating to other specialties has to be done efficiently and quickly. I highly respect the surgical residents for working as hard as they do. It is one thing to work that hard for a month; it is quite another to do it for five years straight. My month in the surgical intensive care unit went very well. I ran through the gauntlet and was found standing on the other side.

Chapter 15: The Oncology Ward

My second sub-internship was a wards month which consisted of covering the floor work on a particular service and learning to be a good intern. I selected the oncology service to see the medicine side of treating cancer since I assumed that I would surgically treat many cancers in my career. Cancer can be one of the most depressing aspects of medicine, but I can't hide from the pain in my patients' lives. The first couple of days consisted of the usual confusion trying to learn about numerous patients that were already on the service. Some of them had been there for over a week with very complicated histories.

The first thing I learned about the oncology service is that it was primarily taking care of previously diagnosed cancer patients with complications. I had envisioned diagnosing cancer and admitting patients for chemotherapy treatment. Now don't get me wrong: there was plenty of this as well, it just wasn't the majority. I guess it was better for my training anyway, less of a focus on hundreds of chemo agents I will never use and more of a focus on medical management of sick patients.

My patient, an elderly man diagnosed with lymphoma, had been admitted for pneumonia and nearly died. He and his daughter were both very pleasant people whom I enjoyed getting to know. Although I'm sure that my youthful appearance could have made her apprehensive, she trusted me with all of her questions, never once giving me a feeling of inadequacy or incompetency, something very important for a young doctor.

Actually, at our very first meeting, I was preparing to do an arterial blood draw on her father. I was a little nervous after having had a couple of unsuccessful attempts in the SICU, but I allowed her to stay in the room while I worked. An arterial draw is slightly more complicated than venous with the possibility of multiple sticks or bleeding.

To my surprise, I got the sample on my first attempt. I then realized most of my difficulty in the SICU was that the patients were very swollen and edematous. As I withdrew the needle, however, blood squirted out and splattered the white bed sheets. Then, when my needle also dripped some blood, I knew I would have to apply pressure with my left hand and risk losing the sample. Luckily, the daughter quickly gloved up to apply pressure for me. Since this specific type of arterial draw is for measuring blood gases, exposing them to the atmosphere for too long would have compromised the results.

I had noticed the patient's frequent confusion, so before I left I asked his daughter about his mental status changes. A million things could cause this in the hospital setting but a few serious ones were on our radar. Apparently, before I started on this service, his oxygen levels had dropped temporarily to dangerous levels. His bout with pneumonia could have deprived his brain of the necessary amount of oxygen. He also could have had a delayed bleed in his brain from a vague history of falling before his admission. A CT scan of his head was negative, but the tricky part of the human body is that the brain can begin bleeding days after the insult, proving again that nothing is ever easy in medicine.

The patient's daughter agreed to give me a report after observing him during their visit, so I left my name and pager number with the nurses. Soon the nurses began paging me instead of the residents for medical questions. It was the first time nurses and family members were calling me for answers, and it felt good. When the daughter paged me to report, she also fired off a laundry list of questions. Luckily, I had spent a lot of time reading about his complicated hospital course beforehand, so I was able to give her a frank assessment. Her sincere appreciation reminded me how important it is to be available and accessible for questions. This was another example of the lessons learned in fourth year.

My second patient, a lung cancer patient with metastases to the brain, exemplifies this as well. I had finished my day, was walking out the door to go home, when I received the page to admit him. Admitting a patient to the hospital is a long, drawn-out process, mainly because we need to log into the computer a complete history and physical. Orders also have to be placed, but this is usually the job of the residents. Even though I was twenty years his junior, he never stopped calling me "doctor" or "sir." I knew he deserved more than to be rushed through the process. Unfortunately, smoking, his one weakness was going to kill him long before he should have died.

The week before his admittance, he had had radiation therapy to try to kill a brain lesion, only to develop severe balance and vision problems. He was here for treatment to decrease the inflammation in his brain in order to restore some of his function. Generally, treatment such as this restores some but not all function. I simply hoped we could get him to the point of being able to walk with a walker. Shortly thereafter, I had to leave town, but I heard we transferred him after a few days to a rehab facility.

Many more patients I met that week touched me in some way. While smoking can cause premature death, working on that perfect tan can be just as deadly. Melanoma, a skin cancer that usually develops from too much sun radiation, has to be about the worst, especially since it can strike younger patients. We had two female patients on our service, a young mother in her 20s, not much older than I, and one in her 30s, with metastatic melanoma. The young mother's cancer had spread so badly that her bones were breaking.

The treatment we were trying was so dangerous that they were both in the ICU, usually vomiting or having significant drops in blood pressure and heart rate. In fact, this treatment was actually a follow-up after the failure of conventional therapies, so we debated the safety and wisdom of another dose, especially since the treatment was not tremendously effective. Despite their extreme level of violent sickness, whenever we decided to go ahead with the next dose, they were relieved. It was their last hope.

During rounds with the whole team we stopped at one of the elderly female patients with metastatic breast cancer who had actually been admitted for breathing problems. Obviously, her appearance was very important to her. If she weren't wearing a wig, she had a hair net to hide her hair loss. Make-up applied, she had fake eyebrows painted on, always looking prim and proper. After numerous nebulizer treatments produced little improvement, we prescribed steroid treatment to decrease inflammation in the lungs. When she refused treatment, we quickly ascertained that her refusal was cosmetic, as her earlier prednisone treatments had caused substantial swelling. "Cancer just takes everything from you," she stated. With a little nudging, we were able to convince her of the importance of taking the medication.

Allow me to digress from the typical patient care stories to describe an important part of the medical school experience. After my first year of med school, I had decided to take it upon myself to perform some clinical research. I didn't know what I wanted to specialize in at that time, so I picked a project in the cardiovascular surgery department that sounded interesting.

I worked with a surgeon who specialized in diseases of the aorta and aortic valve. His particular interest was patients with bicuspid aortic valves (BAV), a congenital defect in which only two leaflets of the heart valve form instead of three. A recent link had been discovered between this type of heart valve and aneurysms of the ascending aorta, the largest artery that comes off the heart. Aneurysms lead to eventual dissection and sudden death. I looked at the patient charts of every person who had their aortic valve replaced from 1990 to 2000, building a database of the patients who had a documented BAV. I found that while only approximately fifty patients had fulfilled the requirements of our study, we knew that some had just not been documented or recorded as judiciously as needed. After all, who would have thought back then that a link such as this would be discovered?

After finding the fifty patients who had BAV, I then undertook the task of calling these former patients, ten to fifteen years after surgery, in order to explain the nature of this research. Some received the news with apprehension while others weren't even vaguely interested in follow-up care. Unfortunately, I couldn't reach the vast majority; and after working for two years, I convinced only twenty to come back to Loyola for a follow-up CT scan of the chest. For the others, I would have thought that a potential life-saving follow-up exam would outweigh the inconvenience of the trip.

I became discouraged a number of times, but with the prodding of my attending, I reached the 20 mark. Remarkably, of the twenty patients, eight (40%) had an ascending aorta classifiable as aneurysmal, an astounding result much higher than anticipated. Of course, the study wasn't perfect since it wasn't a very large study, which decreases the validity of the results, but it was still a significant finding. I submitted the completed abstract to an aortic symposium held at Yale University Medical School. A few weeks later it was accepted as a poster display, a huge honor that I excitedly shared with my supervising heart surgeon. We quickly began work on a six-feet by three-foot medical poster that we barely finished by the deadline.

Making me feel a bit like royalty, the CV surgery department sponsored my flight to the two-day symposium as well as my lodging. At the same time, however, I was nervous about presenting my research to a large group of heart surgeons who knew much more about the heart than I ever would. The symposium was dedicated to John Ritter, the beloved actor who died suddenly from aortic dissection. His widow, well-known actress Amy Yasbeck, was there with their daughter, not only to present a beautiful tribute to her late husband but to also lend her support to research into the aorta. Her speech was quite moving and full of passion as she described her husband's untimely death, which sadly happened on their daughter's fifth birthday. What a tragedy to have to explain to a child.

Although aortic surgery is not going to be my field of interest, it was very worthwhile to see how symposiums are held; proving that the seemingly tedious drill of research could make a difference in the lives of millions of people.

Reality struck again upon my return from Yale as I had to refocus on oncology to finish strongly. We were slammed with patients the first day back, mainly because of the other services' consideration in not consulting us over the weekend. Two of my patients that week developed deep vein thromboses (DVTs), dangerous clots that can break off and travel to the lungs. These clots, called pulmonary emboli, can be lethal.

I was able to make this diagnosis with one of the two patients I picked up upon my return from Yale. During my exam, I noticed that one leg was more swollen than the other. When a Doppler confirmed our suspicions, the patient was started on a blood thinner. The other patient's morbid obesity prevented the same kind of diagnosis. The pain in the leg was there, but the large amount of fat hid any noticeable swelling. However, her complaint of pain in one leg led me to notice that one leg was warmer than the other. The next day she was transferred off our service so it's good that the etiology of her pain was discovered before she was lost in the shuffle. Thinking for myself and making a quick decision gave me a proud feeling.

During my second week, a patient with a sarcoma of the maxillary sinus just below the left eye became my first head-and-neck oncologic patient. Her records indicated that she had had surgery thirty years earlier to remove a benign growth in that area, the same type of procedure that I had recently scrubbed in on during my ENT rotation. Wondering if she were predisposed for cancer in the future, I recalled the poor morbidity that can be caused by cancer of the head. Displacing her eye upward, a large tumor protruded from her cheek, continuing to grow under her scalp and wrapping around her skull. Tumor removal had been discounted since she would have lost not only half her face but her eye as well. The tumor was unresectable. At this point, her only hope of recovery, or at least an extension of survival, rested in chemotherapy. In fact, this was actually her second round of chemo. After learning that the tumor had shrunk slightly from the first round, I wondered what she looked like before the treatment.

Her hospital course was unremarkable for the most part. We gave her every anti-nausea drug in the book, which helped her combat the expected vomiting and diarrhea that accompany chemo. Every morning she ate breakfast without difficulty. My attending described it best, remarking that she was on autopilot, leaving us with very little to do. All of the medications were in a protocol ordered by her primary oncologist upon admission.

I've already mentioned the IL-2 therapy for metastatic melanoma. We treated a lot of them at Loyola. I followed one patient in the medical intensive care unit for the entire week where she didn't get too sick, but we had to constantly monitor her urine output and blood pressure. This patient was young, only in her forties, which reiterates the tragedy of this type of cancer. The tumor had spread to her liver, lungs, and abdomen which translates into a death sentence for most people. However, about fifteen percent of patients respond to this treatment and go into remission. Although she was completely exhausted by the end of the week, everyone involved in her care was encouraged by some shrinkage of her tumors after the first round. We were delighted that she got all of her scheduled doses since patients usually get worse every round. We discharged her to her home, but she would have to come back in a couple of weeks for another week of IL-2.

Halfway through the week I took my first overnight call on the service. I had taken call quite a few times before but this one was going to be a little different. Since I was a sub-intern, the seniors decided to hold me to it. They tagged me with the intern all night and had me carry the on-call pager. For the first time in my life I was being paged by nurses for questions on medication orders as well as by patients with deteriorating symptoms. Of course, the intern was right next to me the entire time, but it was still nerve-wracking.

The first call was from a nurse on the oncology service regarding a patient in rigors, or shaking chills, caused in this patient from a reaction to a platelet transfusion. "I need 25 of Demerol for a patient in rigors." I told her to hold on while I checked with the intern. He didn't seem sure at first, so I told her that we would look at the patient's chart and call her back. "No, I need to give her something now; she's miserable," she responded. The intern had to get on the phone so it wasn't a great success for my first call. For me, this type of wake-up call reminded me that, in only seven months, I would be at the receiving end of the pager with no intern to bail me out. Although senior residents are always available, we are expected to be able to handle most of the calls at night.

We decided to go see the patient. The intern, only one year ahead of me, seemed cool and collected, handling the situation with effective questions and answers. After a new set of vitals showed a dangerously low blood oxygen level, he ordered some oxygen via nasal cannula. In the meantime, she was breathing very rapidly with a look of panic in her eyes. She clearly thought she was going to die. "If I have a seizure," she said, gasping between breaths, "I want you to resuscitate me. I know I'm DNR (do not resuscitate) but I want to be resuscitated." After medication and the discontinuation of blood products, she was fine.

My intern experience taught me that any sojourn at the nurses' station invited constant questions. I mean no disrespect at all for nurses since they are only doing their job and doing it well. Once, during our patient checks away from the station, the nurses paged us with questions every thirty seconds. We finally had to instruct them to save their questions until we returned when we could answer all their questions at one time. I found that I enjoyed the responsibility; it gave me a taste of the residency that was to come.

That week the Angel of Death visited the Oncology Department, claiming the lives of many of our patients. The first one was a female breast cancer patient with a metastasis to the liver that caused the abdomen to flood with fluid. No amount of tapping could stop the fluid build-up. I had noticed on a previous rounding that the usual pre-death confusion had already begun to set in. She was dead within forty-eight hours.

The second patient was the nice man, my patient with balance issues I had mentioned earlier. I actually learned of his passing after my day off when I asked the residents where he was. Their reply that he had been transferred to the eighth floor was clear enough: Loyola has only seven.

I was stunned. I couldn't believe it. He was such a kind person. The oncology fellow took it pretty hard as well, mentioning several times that day that she couldn't believe he was gone. Before his death, he had returned to Loyola where we were shocked by his appearance, describing him best with the word "toxic," the term used in medicine with no specific definition that is more of a gut check when dealing with a seriously ill patient. His impending death had been apparent to him, too, as he cried that cold Saturday morning, using a handkerchief to dry away the tears. That image of him has been superimposed in my mind. We were moved by his sadness, only barely managing a "hang in there" as we left the room.

Three other deaths occurred that week, one patient in the bone marrow transplant unit and two in the pediatric unit. Death is not the only tragedy that happened during my last week on oncology. One elderly cancer patient with the common complication of clotting disorder presented to the ER with a cold hand that subsequently had to be amputated. Afterward she was transferred to our service for management. Cancer makes the blood clot easier and needs intensive medical management. While her stump was well treated and wrapped, she still cried from the pain. To make matters worse, her son was quite difficult. When we entered the room on rounds, he was livid about a blood thinner medication that had been added after being discontinued two weeks prior. He ranted about the cost of the medication, arguing to the attending that "it's still probably less than what you make in a day." We already suspected him of neglecting his mother, whose poor hygiene left little to the imagination. Her medical file had notations of suspected abuse as well. The son wanted to keep her at home, most likely to receive funding for her care, using the term "care" loosely. Unfortunately, suspicion was not enough, so we let the social workers do their job and discharged her home.

One of the saddest situations of the entire month involved a middle-aged woman ravaged by colon cancer. Her wasted condition told the tale of imminent death, a fact confirmed by lab values. We notified the immediate family, only to learn that she had no husband or parents, just two teenage children, the older an 18-year-old daughter who would have to be the decision maker. Both of them were extremely upset by the misunderstanding that we would no longer care for her since death was certain. We reassured them that we would care for her and make her as comfortable as possible, but that any other treatment would be an act of futility. These two kids were alone with their dying mother. She was so near death by this time she could barely speak. The end was coming, and coming within days.

She died early one morning while we were on rounds. Due to some miscommunication, the message wasn't relayed to us for over half an hour, and the family was upset that a physician had not come right away. As we approached the room, the attending sent the responsible intern in to deal with the problem he had created. By the time we apologized for the situation, the family had already entered the grieving phase and could care less about our explanations. With the teenagers in tears around the bed, I looked at the lifeless figure before me. Sometimes the dead appear more at peace than in their final moments. It was true in her case. It's as if the struggling has ended and they can finally rest. With her passing, the week of death on the oncology service came to a close.

On my second call night, we were in the intensive care unit rounding on our IL-2 melanoma patients, who weren't doing so well. A young mother in her early thirties had just been diagnosed with leukemia in the ER, so, as one can imagine, she was quite hysterical. Having suffered with cold-like symptoms and night sweats for a few months, her primary care physician sent her to Loyola ER after he saw the results of the blood tests. Our repeat blood test showed too many blast cells, immature white blood cells that shouldn't be seen in the circulation. They should be growing into normal immune cells in the bone marrow. In her case, a baby immune cell had spun out of control and divided millions of times to form an army of clones.

As we walked into her room she was lying on the bed with her husband. Her parents were standing at the side of the bed, and they all were crying. They sat up immediately as the resident introduced us. We informed her that she would be admitted to the hematology service for immediate treatment. A bone marrow biopsy in the morning would give more information as to the type of cancer. "Please tell me this is a dream and I'm going to wake up!" she cried as she buried her face in her hands. The family rushed to her side and cried with her. I felt the onset of tears in my eyes and quickly fought against showing any emotion.

"Detach," I told myself for my own sanity. She wanted to know how much time she had left, but we had no answer to give her. Then she asked to see her baby before being admitted to the service as she would be in-house for a month getting treatment, making her susceptible to infections. A common virus healthy people shrug off can kill an immunocompromised patient. Nothing about this situation was good. The following morning one of the hematology residents told me that she had just left the patient's room, the entire family weeping as the reality of the situation replaced the initial shock. The resident broke down and cried with them.

I see pain all the time at work, but I still couldn't imagine the pain they were experiencing. That same day we sent home one of the IL-2 patients because she was too sick from the treatment. She didn't finish her doses. Whether or not the melanoma would eventually take her life depended on the last few doses she received. I wished her the best of luck. I wished all of the oncology patients I met that month the best of luck. They were inspiring individuals, maintaining composure and strength in the face of the ultimate adversity. They taught me a lot about being a good physician. For one thing, it is perfectly normal to empathize with suffering patients. The key is to keep it from interfering with your work.

When I finished my oncology rotation I was more excited than I had been in a long time to enjoy my scheduled month of vacation time. Although my intentions were to devote the time to interviewing and studying for Step 2 of the boards, in reality, I spent much of the time doing some serious resting and relaxing. The most difficult rotations of fourth year were finally over. The following semester would be much more low-key. I looked forward to the electives as I felt they would broaden my skills as a physician and make me a better doctor in the long run.

Chapter 16: Emergency Medicine

The emergency department has undergone a variety of changes over the past few decades. With the advent of the new specialty of Emergency Medicine, the field has evolved into a more homogenous blend of physicians. Whereas the departments used to be staffed by Internal Medicine, Family Practice and General Surgeons, now most physicians are board certified in Emergency Medicine. Only the most rural departments are still staffed by other specialties and then only out of necessity.

With the recent changes in board certification, citizens across the country now have 24-hour-a-day access to quick and life-saving care. Depending on to whom one speaks this is both good and bad. With legislative involvement, such laws as EMTALA have made it illegal to turn down care to any individual under any circumstance. The 24-hour-a-day access to emergency care has since developed into free care for the uninsured people of our country, citizen and non-citizen alike. Not that providing care is a bad thing; it is simply an economical and controversial problem.

Emergency departments across the country suffer from money shortages and closures, the problem stemming from the large number of uninsured people in our country using them as primary care clinics. Anything from simple upper respiratory tract infections to chronic headaches often jam the overcrowded departments and delay life-saving care to those who need it. Emergency Medicine physicians have to perform expensive workups on these patients to rule out the rare but serious diseases that can arise. The malpractice issue plays a huge role in this practice of "safety medicine." Because deadly disease can masquerade in a simple, atypical form in the ED, EM physicians have experienced the full frontal assault of trial lawyers across the country. It turns into a cascading, downward spiral.

During my rotation at Loyola's Emergency Department, these problems were obvious. Most staff workers couldn't remember a time in recent history when the hospital was so congested, with long waits and a slow pace that affected the patients. With the recent closure of dozens of Cook County clinics, the underserved populations in Chicago were herded into the free emergency departments in the area. It was a catalyst to the already burdened EDs in the area, fast-forwarding the tumultuous problems decades ahead in time. While the problems with the Emergency Department in our society will not be resolved over night, one fact still holds true: Emergency Medicine cannot be scrutinized because lives are being saved on a daily basis in EDs across the country. At least we have that to say about our often criticized healthcare system.

After a five week break for residency interviews, I began my month a little rusty, mainly because my mind was still on vacation. I couldn't get myself to work as hard as these physicians are used to seeing so it was a difficult first week. Spending too much time on the computer earned me a firm but diplomatic scolding, but I was soon back on track because of it. I wanted to do an ER elective so I could sharpen my differential and diagnostic skills prior to entering internship. I saw a wide range of disorders ranging from benign to acute in severity. Of course, I also snatched up the patients that presented something related to ENT since I will be consulted in my residency as a specialist to see these types of patients in the ED. I figured I would get a head start and see how they are worked up by the ER docs.

In addition to the grind of the ER, I spent one day at the Illinois poison control center in downtown Chicago. I listened to phone conversations as the toxicology specialists answered questions on everything from scared mothers calling about their toddlers to Emergency Physicians around the state inquiring about overdose treatment for a patient of theirs. It was a good experience and a nice change of pace from the typical patient care setting.

My first patient of the entire month was a nose bleeder. One may consider that trivial, but people die all the time from nosebleeds. A huge portion of the population live on blood thinners for a variety of reasons, which makes controlling bleeds more difficult. I couldn't see much on the exam due to the blood. Consequently, I had little information to offer the attending when I presented. As soon as he heard I had a bleeder, he ran and grabbed some neosynephrine to squirt in the guy's nose. Neosynephrine is a vasoconstrictor and, with a little pressure, will control most bleeds. Over the counter Afrin will do the same thing.

After the bleeding is stopped, one simply packs the nose to prevent future bleeds. In difficult cases, a thin strip of white material similar to a tampon is guided through the nose. Saline is then sprayed on the strip causing a dramatic expansion, completely sealing off the nostril. We took a more simple approach with a combination approach of Surgicell and lubrication.

Although I didn't see as much ENT pathology as I would have liked, I did see a complicated ear infection, but there is not much one can do in the ER except to prescribe antibiotics and pain killers. This gentleman had allowed an infection to worsen for weeks, and now suffered from excruciating pain. Severe tenderness to the bone immediately behind the ear caused me to suspect mastoiditis, a severe complication with ear infections. The bacteria had spread to the bone behind the ear and were only millimeters away from the brain. He was given antibiotics and scheduled for surgery with ENT. They drilled him a few days later.

It never ceases to amaze me how much I still have to learn about medicine to even look competent. My next patient, a pleasant elderly female patient, had experienced little urine output over the previous day, the low output caused by her "Indiana pouch." As many of us do in the medical profession, I Googled for a two-minute lesson, learning that her bladder had been surgically removed because of cancer. Part of her colon was then shaped and molded into a new bladder with a created tract leading to her abdomen. During scheduled periods throughout the day, she inserted a catheter through her abdomen into the Indiana pouch to urinate. This quick tutorial allowed me to ask the right questions during exam in the ED. My confidence at least gave the appearance of education and knowledge of her medical and surgical history. I think it was best that she was not made aware of the fact that I knew nothing of her condition a few minutes before.

During the interview, someone in the next exam room went into a convulsive seizure, prompting a boisterous, organized chaos that actually distracted me a bit. My patient remained quite calm and continued to tell me her complaints. She was admitted to the urology service for further care, and I had no further contact. This is the main reason I didn't go into Emergency Medicine. Many acute care patients are transferred to another service, resulting in a lost doctor-patient relationship that barely even started. I want to be the specialist taking care of the patients both surgically and medically. I did, however, look up as many patients as I could remember to see what eventually happened to them. The ER docs encouraged me to do this as well to further my educational experience.

As the month progressed I continued to improve my presentations and my time in the exam rooms. Emergency is all about continuous history and physicals on patients never seen before. Since the waiting rooms are usually jam-packed, this must be done quickly, an executed philosophy somewhat callously referred to as moving meat. Rarely would I get floored by a patient and not know what to do, yet this happened during my second week. I walked into the room to see a young, teenage boy lying on the bed, surrounded by his somewhat distraught family. I introduced myself as usual and asked the young guy what brought him in today. Without saying a word, he lifted his left hand and silently tapped on his head. After a moment of perplexity, his mother interrupted with the story. He had just been diagnosed with a brain tumor. The family wanted to see Neurosurgery.

Although I was stunned by the information, I still had no idea why they came to the ER. Even though brain tumors are quite serious, they can usually be handled on an outpatient basis. I had to ascertain whether they were sent here by their physician or if they simply panicked from the information. I decided to perform a complete history and physical as if he were a standard patient. He described having had a severe headache for two weeks, accompanied by balance problems. His primary care doctor had ordered a brain scan, sending them to the ER that same day. I couldn't discern any neurological abnormalities on examination. When I presented to my attending, he was just as unsure as I was as to why they were in the ED. Luckily, they had brought the MRI films which gave the answer. The tumor was causing his brain to slowly herniate through the bottom of his skull.

He needed decompressive surgery as soon as possible. We soon discovered that everything had already been arranged between the primary doctor and the neurosurgery team. A simple call to the ED staff would have prevented much confusion, not to mention saving the patient from a complete neurological examination that would be repeated by the neurosurgical resident a few minutes later. He was carted off by the brain surgeons, and they did their work. I wish now I had asked to accompany them since the ER docs probably wouldn't have minded. Although it was unnecessary, my examining a patient like that is a rare learning experience. The fact that I didn't pick up on anything on my exam probably meant that I needed to work on it. About midway through my rotation, I had accomplished many of my goals pertaining to diagnostics, but I lacked some procedural experience. Although it sounds morbid, I began to hunt for cases to practice on, figuring the best case scenario is to practice with physician supervision before my residency.

As an ENT I will be responsible for facial trauma call, sewing up major facial lacerations all by myself. Sure, I will always be able to call for help, but part of being a successful physician is being effective. That week, I got a couple of nice "lacs," the first guy having punched through a window after arguing with his girlfriend. He had a jagged cut with visible muscle and tendon that needed some special suturing. An x-ray was performed to make sure no glass was left in the wound prior to closure. In order to pull the lac together and stabilize it, the ER doc taught me a special "dog ears" knot that involved looping the needle underneath the skin and lassoing the jagged edge together.

The next lac was on a tough old gal, an elderly female who had slammed her finger in the car door. Her husband brought her in when the bleeding hadn't stopped. I first asked her about any medications, most specifically blood thinners, and wasn't surprised when she said she was on Coumadin, which explained the profuse bleeding. A far cry from the tough young man I had just sutured, she adamantly refused any pain medication. Before sewing, I numbed her finger with lidocaine, inserting the needle into the skin adjacent to the wound and delivering some medication. I had to make sure all areas were numb so I pushed the needle all the way across her finger, accidentally sending it out the other side. Luckily, the lidocaine had already begun working, so she didn't feel much. I brought it back a little, injected a little more medication, and then repeated the process on the other side of the wound. I finished the job quickly, and the bleeding stopped immediately.

My good luck with procedures prompted me to branch it out a bit. I noticed a powerfully-built young patient, early twenties, with extreme dental pain, giving me a pain rating of ten-out-of-ten. I figured I might get some of these complaints as an ENT, even though it is closer to the dental realm. I decided this would be a good time to practice my first nerve block. A local injection of lidocaine above the tooth would completely alleviate the pain, allowing time for the patient to schedule an appointment with a dentist. Similarly, I could inject the needle below the eye and completely numb the entire area, leaving the specific method up to the attending. I broke out the textbooks and quickly read about the procedure. The attendings picked up on my enthusiasm and taught me as much as they could.

After all of my preparation, I went to tell the patient about my plans, certain he could handle a little needle stick. Wincing like a scared child, he adamantly rejected my idea and settled for pain medication instead, completely destroying any hope I had of practicing a nerve block. Dejected, I told the attending the news, and they wrote the script. At least I learned about the procedural steps so I would be ready if another chance came along.

After I had my fun with procedures, the ED went through a boring spell. The hospital had been so congested for days on end that the hospital went on bypass, the ED refusing to take any transfers or patients via ambulance. Only those patients who brought themselves were seen, so, while the hospital stayed very busy, the ED slowed tremendously. As soon as hospital beds opened up, we came off bypass for a few hours, only to return to it as soon as the hospital filled. This went on for a significant portion of my rotation. Most of the patients I saw were primary care, including one guy who came in at 3 AM for new onset phlegm in his throat. Why in the world would anyone waste hours at the ED in the middle of the night for such a complaint? It never ceases to amaze me.

I'm not saying that exciting emergencies do not occur. In the middle of the night one of the ER docs and I were chatting when a page came overhead, "ER doctor to room 3." We quickly ran to the room to see a rather large woman lying on the bed, completely surrounded by nurses. Having been stripped naked by the staff, she stared at the ceiling, completely unresponsive. This was a true emergency. We jumped into action getting as much data as we could from the paramedics. The only information we had was that she had been drinking excessively with her friend before collapsing. A mention of an empty prescription bottle in her purse began floating around.

During exam, I looked into her empty eyes, my mind reeling. Multiple etiologies began popping into my differential: alcohol or drug overdose, bleed in the brain from hitting her head, hypoglycemic coma, heart attack or arrhythmia, stroke. The ER doc can't miss anything and often has little to go on.

A battery of tests was initiated. After it was set in motion, I left the room to check on my other patients. After some time had passed, I went back to check on her. "You missed all of the fun," the nurses told me as I entered the room. Foul-smelling vomit covered the patient and the floor below, soaking her hair and the sheets below her. I decided to help the nurses clean up. She was a heavy individual, and they needed help rolling her to change the sheets. The vomit wafted a distinct aroma of alcohol. One of the nurses was convinced she knew the exact brand from the vomit's aroma. I didn't know whether to congratulate her on her newfound skill or politely laugh. I decided on both.

When it came time for my shift's end, I passed her onto another resident. With the combination of cramming for Step Two of the boards, transitioning from days to nights and then back to days, I was completely overwhelmed the last two weeks of my elective. Consequently, I neglected to check on her diagnosis, chiding myself for missing an important part of training.

One quite memorable case involved a patient with an excruciating headache. Keeping track of the number of headache complaints that come to the ED is impossible. The vast majority of them are completely benign, making it very easy to cast off their symptoms as nothing more than a tension or migraine headache. Still, missing the rare, serious problems can be catastrophic. My patient was another young guy in high school, very overweight, presenting with a one-day history of headache.

It was the worst headache he ever had, worse on the right side of his skull. Finally deciding on a head scan, we discovered nothing more than "mildly dilated ventricles." This finding could be a normal variant or it could be the beginning signs of pressure build-up in the skull or meningitis. Many lethal diseases were now on our differential. We had no other choice but to do a spinal tap.

After procedure prep, we had him lie on his side and curl up in a ball to spread his spinous processes. In order to access the spinal fluid, we had to penetrate the needle in between the spinous processes of the vertebrae. The only problem was his large body habitus. His extreme obesity complicated the procedure by making it much more technically difficult. After numbing his lower back with lidocaine, we penetrated the needle deep into his back, every once in a while stopping to check the needle for clear fluid. It wasn't long before the long needle was completely inserted. We pulled back and tried again with no success.

After a few futile attempts, we realized we were going to be unsuccessful. The next step was to call radiology to perform the tap under fluoroscopic guidance. X-rays would be used to guide the needle into the proper position.

I had the delightful privilege of calling the radiology attending to inform him of the need for his services. The day was about over, and he was extremely ticked off for having to stay late. He let me know it full well by being extremely rude on the phone. In fact, I've never had an attending act so unprofessional. I proudly kept my cool and handled the situation in a very polite manner, even thanking him for his services. Perhaps I am still naïve and the years of training haven't yet embittered me. I later worked next to him on another rotation and quickly learned that he spoke to everyone that way.

Stat labs were drawn and the patient was carted off to the specials lab. I looked him up later and found that his cerebrospinal fluid was normal, no signs of infection or bleeding. The opening pressure was also within normal limits, ruling out a buildup of pressure in the brain. As often happens in medicine, playing it safe caused some temporary pain and hassle in a patient. Nevertheless, putting patients through some discomfort is necessary to avoid missing the one patient with a lethal pathological process.

On another shift, I witnessed another example of the problems facing emergency departments across the country. One extremely bitter cold winter with temperatures plunging below zero, I saw a patient come in with the complaint of frostbite, something that not every medical student gets to see every day. I quickly assigned him to my roster. He must have been homeless: the smell nearly knocked me over when I walked into the room. His clothes were covered in dirt and he had all of his earthly possessions with him. Although I felt compassion for him, I struggled with conflicting thoughts concerning the validity of his complaints. His hands and feet were covered with black spots with the skin peeling in certain areas. He reported that the pain was so severe he could barely put his shoes on. When I tried to examine them, he hollered in pain and pushed me away.

I had thought this would be a simple slam dunk case with a valuable learning point. Uncertain about a diagnosis, I decided to go in with the attending to watch how someone more experienced would handle the situation. When the patient tried the same maneuver during examination, the attending held his feet and examined him anyway. I learned that the patient has to be examined in spite of complaints of severe pain. I needed to be more confident and gutsy, something that can still be done with compassion.

"Are you hungry?" the attending asked. "We'll get you a sandwich and let you rest here tonight." After we left the room, he told me the plan. We would feed him and, if he stayed until the morning, we would have social work find him a temporary place to stay. Loyola would absorb the cost of his visit. It could range from hundreds to thousands of dollars lost with each visit. Due to the current legislation, patients cannot be turned away even if their complaint is not legitimate. They can be discharged after a thorough evaluation but not prior. Luckily, the department wasn't busy that night so it didn't deprive any other sick patients from being seen.

Later I went to check on him and to get some more information. On the streets for most of his life, he admitted to having schizophrenia. He did stay at a homeless shelter, but he often avoided it because he couldn't tolerate the people there. Often people with schizophrenia have difficulty in social situations and prefer to be alone, even if it means facing the bitter cold of the windy city. He hadn't even bothered to remove an old, dirty hospital band on his wrist from a different Chicago hospital. He bounced from hospital to hospital for food and shelter from the cold. It is a drain on the healthcare system, but there is no easy solution.

As I was wrapping up my rotation in Emergency Medicine, most of my attention was on the upcoming board examination I needed to pass in order to become a physician. One last patient encounter left an impression on me. A page was announced overhead for an attending to come to room two. By this time I had learned that it was usually something serious when that happened. Since two nearby attendings rushed into the room, I resumed typing my note since the room already appeared crowded. Another attending peeked in and said, "This might be something you want to see."

I rushed into the room to see the unconscious, heaving patient breathing laboriously and spraying blood out of his nose, splattering both attendings, the floor, and the curtain at the other end of the room. Estimating his age to be in the mid-thirties, I learned that his father had brought him in after he had collapsed. A blood-pressure monitor showed his pressures to be elevated to an emergent level. I watched the two attendings examine him in their blood-splattered coats. I later learned that a nurse had tried to insert a breathing tube through the nose, causing a nosebleed, a good example of how easy it is to get distracted down a wrong diagnostic track in an emergency situation. Although the bleeding was dramatic, it had nothing to do with the underlying pathology.

While the patient was intubated to assist his breathing, I was directed to find the father and gather more information. I found him talking to the receptionist so I asked him to come to a quieter area and tell me what happened. To my dismay, I couldn't understand his strong, rapid accent and my asking him to repeat things several times resulted in his extreme annoyance. Nevertheless, I reported what information I could get to the attending. As he was prepared for CT scan, the attending and I had the task of telling the father the critical news. Since his son was no longer breathing on his own, he was placed on life-support. With the situation so grave, he should call the rest of the family.

Since his son had had a multitude of medical problems in the past, the father just assumed that this trip would be a simple tune up. He was clearly floored with the information, never suspecting the situation to be as serious as it was. As he left to call his wife, the physician and I went back to work on our other patients. The attending placed the crisis in the back of her mind as she checked on critical lab values for other patients. I tried to do likewise but found it difficult to get the situation out of my head. Less than twenty minutes later, I pulled up the CT scan of his head, realizing the prognosis almost immediately. A large bleed was present, and his brain was beginning to distort from compression.

"Is that his CT?" another attending asked. "Yeah, he's a goner." Neurosurgery came quickly to evaluate him for emergency surgery. Sometimes the skull can be drilled open to drain the blood and relieve the pressure. By this time, more family had arrived to discuss their options. However, as the patient was transferred out of the emergency department, his vitals began to drop. His brain began to herniate through the bottom of his skull. Everyone knew the impending consequence. Before intervention could be carried out, he breathed his last and died.

Chapter 17: Pathology

Pathology is a far cry from ENT, but I wanted to see a side of medicine I had little exposure to. I also had plans to gear the elective to my advantage. Pathology is the field of medicine that performs autopsies, looks at surgical specimens for diagnosis, and handles many of the lab tests administered in the hospital. Every time a specimen is removed surgically, it is sent to pathology. The pathologists decide with the aid of the microscope whether a mass is cancer and if the surgical margins are clean. They are the specialists of the human cell, using special stains and machines to determine if subtle variations in a microscopic cell make it pathology or not.

When the cause of death is uncertain, an autopsy is performed to investigate. The field is surprisingly diverse ranging from CSI-like medical examiners to academic practice. Many of them do fellowships to specialize further in skin, brain, or any other organ of interest. Some focus only on blood and run the large blood banks in the hospital.

My month focused on the surgical side of the specialty. I wanted to get a great variety of experiences while paying special attention to the head and neck specimens from the local ENTs. A typical day included "grossing" specimens from the previous day's operations, which entails preserving the organ in formalin overnight, not only preserving properties but also making the tissue firmer and easier to cut and be examined. The resident records the observations on a microphone controlled by foot pedals. Not that I want to admit watching the show, but the resident reminded me of Scully on *The X-Files*.

The first morning I saw everything from a stomach to a large prostate tumor. After grossing for a couple of hours, the resident and I went to the lounge to look at slides from the specimens she had grossed the day before.

176

In the meantime, the lab technicians make slides from the appropriate samples by encasing them in a medium and using a machine to make tiny cuts much smaller than a human hair. Before the process is finished, sample slides are made from all corners of the sample. Cancer could be ruled in or ruled out and the margins could be declared clean or positive for cancer. If cancer had invaded the margins, the prognosis for the patient was much worse. The surgeon would either have to go back in to take more tissue or the patient referred to an oncologist for chemotherapy or radiation.

After going over the slides, the resident wrote the reports just as she would do in private practice, later going over them again with the attending to double check her work. The process was tedious, but the only safe way to learn. When we signed out the slides to the attending, we went into a room equipped with large microscopes placed around a table to allow us to view the exact image the attending saw. Every now and then she zoomed into a certain area and asked us both questions regarding the specific cells we were viewing. I found it interesting for the first hour, but then I began daydreaming with my eyes firmly fixed into the microscope.

On my first day the on-call team allowed me to tag along for my first autopsy experience. Most of the autopsies in the hospital setting are on extremely sick patients making the cause of death difficult to ascertain. I had watched videos of autopsies during my first two years of medical school but had never witnessed one on an adult before. In fact, although I had completely dissected a corpse in gross anatomy, the process somehow seemed less humane on a fresh body. As we ventured to the hospital's basement morgue, I remembered the autopsy on the baby during my pediatric rotation. I got completely suited up in a gown, face shield, and gloves as the autopsy technician prepared the body, an elderly female who had serious medical problems. Her sudden death prompted the distraught family to ask for an autopsy.

To begin, we made basic observations about her body size and habitus. Recent surgery had left a fresh, abdominal incision that leaked a brown, foul-smelling liquid. Her mannequin-like legs were pearly white, very edematous and freezing to the touch. When the okay was given, the technician pushed a button, and water began to flow underneath the table to carry away the bodily fluids. The residents primarily watched the technician's flurry of activity and made observations. He made a large, U-shaped incision on the chest and peeled the skin away. The incision was carried down the abdomen to open it up completely. An accidental nick in the small intestine caused the intestinal contents to spill out, presenting an odor far worse than anything I had ever experienced in gross anatomy class. He then used a saw to open the chest cavity, removing the sternum and the front portions of the ribs to reveal the heart and lungs.

After the trachea and esophagus were cut, the entire chest and abdominal viscera were pulled out in one gigantic mass of tissue and handed to residents. While the technician cleaned the shell of the body and sewed up the large incision, I followed the residents to the other table to see how the investigational process would play out. One by one they inspected each organ, then handed each to me to be weighed. The supervising attending showed us the best way to cut open the lungs to find the blood vessels coursing through them for the purpose of checking for a pulmonary embolus, a blood clot traveling from veins in the legs. PE's are a common cause of sudden death in the hospital and have to be considered.

The attending wanted a thorough inspection for recurrence of tumor, almost hoping for evidence of one in order to make the family's earlier decision for DNR easier. I had never thought of cancer recurrence being a comforting factor to a grieving family, but I can follow that logic now. Unfortunately, no cancer was detected, and no single cause could be determined. The family would have to find solace elsewhere.

We grossed specimens and looked at slides the following day. The grossing room was a beehive of activity with a grossly infected colon from a neutropenic patient on the resident's table and a large, amputated leg on another's. Having been amputated above the knee, the leg was black and gangrenous in certain parts, with only three toes remaining as the others had been amputated previously. I knew from my vascular rotation that the patient was diabetic with severe peripheral vascular disease. An embolus had likely put the finishing touches on the once viable leg. As my resident and I grossed the colon, I couldn't help but look back at the leg.

Boggy and covered with green feces, the colon came from an immunocompromised patient, most likely a leukemic patient in the bone marrow transplant intensive care unit. An infection had ravaged the colon without an adequate immune system to respond. I'm sure a heroic attempt of antibiotic use was carried out, but medicine is limited. I had to fish through the surrounding fatty tissue in search of lymph nodes, which always have to be examined to rule out any coinciding cancer. When my resident had to leave to answer a page, the other resident asked if I could stay and help gross the leg. I accepted the offer since it is not every day one holds an amputated leg in his hands.

After the initial measurements were taken, the resident cut deep into the calf muscle in search of the arteries. I held the cold, dead leg hoping he wouldn't slip with his knife and stab me, worrying more when the knife slipped in the other direction. He found the artery quickly, hard as a rock through years of atherosclerotic calcification of the arteries. There was hardly a patent lumen visible to the human eye. Cross sections were taken for further examination. We then headed to the main arteries of the foot for the same type of investigation, making serial slices on top of the foot until we spotted the artery. The usual curiosities creeping into my head, I wondered who the patient was and how he or she was coping with the loss of a leg. My brief stint on vascular was enough to know how hard patients take losing a limb. I suppose no rotation at all is needed for such a realization; just being human is quite enough.

Week two was spent on the cytology service. Any time a fluid is tapped in the body, it is sent to cytology where the specialists focus on microscopic cells smeared onto a slide. Pap smears, spinal tap fluid, and fine-needle aspirations (FNAs) of tumors are just a few examples. The majority of the week was quite boring; however, I had a motive for choosing this sub-specialty. Thyroid nodules or tumors are always evaluated by FNA prior to surgery or medical therapy. The cytology fellows are needed at the bedside of the patients being biopsied to evaluate the smears for adequate cells. I found the perfect opportunity to see my first thyroid FNA. Although most ENTs perform thryoidectomies, many do not have the training to do the FNA for diagnosis.

When we walked into the room, the radiology residents were prepping the patient for the biopsy. Ultrasound was used to identify the enlarged nodule. It was a grainy image, but I found myself beginning to see the anatomy.

After the patient was instructed not to swallow, as swallowing moves the thyroid gland up and down, a large needle was inserted, visible as it pierced into the abnormal nodule. The resident began pumping the needle in and out to remove as many cells as possible. The needle was removed and handed to the cytology fellow. He went into a quick motion of spreading the droplets onto slides and staining them with dyes. Meanwhile, the radiology residents repeated the same procedure on the patient as one needle biopsy is usually inadequate. The fellow taught me how to stain the slides and I did it thereafter. A quick glance under the microscope showed adequate cells and the procedure was finished. Most thyroid nodules are benign, but they have to be evaluated to rule out cancer. This patient was one of the lucky ones.

The most important relationship the surgeons have with the pathologists is the submission of specimens directly from the operating table for frozen evaluation. We call it "sending frozens." Week three of my rotation was spent on-call with the pathology resident performing frozens. She was an intern and graciously allowed me to participate in the process, one which I found to be a bit hectic, as multiple specimens can be sent at once from multiple surgeons, each expecting a fast answer as to the preliminary diagnosis.

It all goes down like this: a small lymph node is removed next to a tumor in the operating room. The surgeon wants to know if the cancer cells have spread to the adjacent lymph nodes, worsening the patient's prognosis. The specimen is tubed directly from the operating room to the pathology laboratory in a completely different building. Once received, the pathologist either takes samples from the specimen or, if small enough, submits the entire sample for frozen analysis.

The lymph node is placed on a small circular device and covered in gel. The apparatus is turned upside down and placed on a frigid metal pane. Spraying the sample with a specialized aerosol causes the gel to immediately freeze, encasing the sample. The next step in the process is to make the slides. The sample is loaded onto a lever that moves up and down with rotation of an external crank. As the sample comes down, a precisely placed blade shaves off a five micrometer slice, which translates to five-millionths of a meter. The thin shave is placed onto a slide and then stained appropriately. This is where my job came into play.

I took the slide from the resident with the nearly invisible cut of lymph node. A panel of stains and alcohol solutions for dehydration was assembled before me, some panels needing only ten dips while others required up to a minute of soaking. An instructional sheet on the wall provided me with the specific instructions. When the process was complete, a quick cover slip was placed to protect the now visible specimen.

At this point, the attending looked at the slide under the microscope, teaching both of us the appropriate lessons from that case. Providing immediate access to the surgeons, a speaker phone related the diagnosis. If there were no significant problems, a diagnosis could be given to the surgeon within twenty minutes of sending the sample. If the lymph node was positive for cancer invasion, the surgeon could then perform the appropriate dissection to increase survival. As samples could come from multiple operating rooms at the same time, the process could become quite stressful. Every pathology resident loves to have a future surgeon rotate on frozens to instill a sense of patience when it comes to receiving a diagnosis.

One frozen case stands out in my mind. After wrapping up a particular case, I turned to see a gigantic container with the next specimen. The resident and I peeled off the covering to see an ovarian cyst the size of a large watermelon, thirty centimeters in diameter and full of fluid. She was an intern and had never had anything like this before; we were equally astonished. Even seasoned pathologists walking by couldn't resist the urge to get a close-up view of our new-found entertainment. I participated in the surgical removal of a large ovarian cyst on my gyn-onc rotation, but I think this particular cyst had that one beaten. The ovary needed to be weighed but no scale in the laboratory was large enough to handle it. We opted to drain the fluid from the cyst and weigh each separately.

The ovary was in a large bucket when we began the process. My resident plunged the scalpel into the cyst and brown fluid resembling chocolate milk began pouring out of the puncture hole. The bucket was half-filled with the fluid but the process not over. We discovered it had multiple loculations, or sacs, containing mucous. Before I could intervene, the resident opened up another sac, producing the same brown fluid. By this time, the bucket was nearly full of the chocolaty solution and began to overflow onto our counter. I quickly grabbed some smaller containers and poured the overflow into them. We filled two other containers before the gushing finally stopped. After the cyst was completely opened, a large number of smaller cysts were seen.

The frozen slides gave a preliminary diagnosis of an ovarian cancer and the permanent slides were made. It was a tedious process as one specimen had to be submitted for every centimeter in diameter. A sample of the nearly obliterated fallopian tube was submitted as well. Cleanup took just about as long since the entire bench was covered with mucous.

Most days of the week were quite slow with momentary accelerations in the pace of things. Only one day of the week was heavy on operations requiring frozens. Since the last day of the week was one of the slow days I decided to tag along with one of the neuropathologists. He invited me to come and watch as he dissected a brain in front of a local high school AP class having recently learned the entire brain anatomy. The pathologist began the dissection with a camera projecting close-ups onto TV monitors. I stood at the side of the class with the teachers, enjoying what I thought would be a nice review of neuroanatomy that I hadn't reviewed in years. I had no idea what was in store for me although I should have seen it coming.

The pathologist began asking me pimp questions about the anatomy and physiology of the brain, half of which I couldn't remember. To add insult to injury, he then asked the questions I didn't know to the class of high schools students, who quite easily answered most of them.

Although I was right on some of the questions, the situation was rather embarrassing for me. The high school students interested in medicine still came up to me afterward to ask questions. I suppose that gives me some satisfaction with the experience. Overall, the field trip had to be quite amazing for the students. After the pathologist filleted the brain into multiple cross-sections, the students gloved up and examined the specimens. I doubt they will forget the anatomy of the brain that they held in their hands anytime soon.

Excluding the pimp session, I really enjoyed talking to younger students about medicine. Perhaps it is something I can do in my future practice. A couple of days later I traveled out to Aurora, Illinois to talk to some fourth graders about medicine. One of my friends is a teacher and thought it would be a good idea to have me come answer any questions they had. Fortunately for me, they didn't stump me. Bringing a few preserved organs with me increased my popularity.

On my final week of the rotation, I spent a lot of time preparing for my final presentation to the pathology department. I found some time for clinical teaching but avoided anything excessive. One day was spent with dermatopathology, looking at slides from moles and other skin lesions, an assembly line of hundreds of slides that hurt my eyes by the end of the day. I also spent a day down in the microbiology laboratory. My goal at this time was to see a few different subspecialties to simply get an idea of what they do. The resident showed me how to grow fungi and other microorganisms isolated from different patients. We took a plate that had grown fungi for a few days, touched it with tape, and then looked at the tape under the microscope. A nearby textbook with pictures aided in our diagnosis.

Next, she wanted to show me how to look at a stool sample. A small container filled with processed stool from a patient with diarrhea was opened. We placed a drop on a large slide followed by some iodine. Under the microscope the view was mostly obscured with unrecognizable debris. I could hardly believe a small drop of stool could cause such an atrocious odor. Perhaps the processing condensed the smell into this one small droplet. At one point we saw in the center of the field, a spiral-like cylinder similar in appearance to a slinky. After quizzing me a few times, she decided to give me the diagnosis: a muscle fiber from the patient's diet. She moved the slide and began pointing out digested vegetation and other artifacts that could confuse a young resident. She finally found the etiology of the diarrhea, a parasite unlike anything I had ever seen before. She made me study its physical structures and skim through the textbook. With some prompting, I made the diagnosis in about ten minutes. Skimming through the book, I realized how many organisms I had never heard of. During my second-year microbiology class, I was certain I learned the majority of them due to how rigorous the class was.

With the advancement of knowledge and science, no one can ever learn it all. Since I had little interest in studying stool under a microscope, that was fine with me. Pathology was over and only two rotations were left. Senioritis began to sink in as I began my Neurology rotation.

Chapter 18: Neurology

Neurology was one of the four-week required rotations of fourth year, a service that takes care of abnormalities of the brain, including strokes and seizures. Spending two weeks each on the wards and consult service, I began with the wards, which mainly housed stroke patients. I was in the company of three other medical students and two residents. Overall, the rotation was not too bad in terms of hours worked. The residents were laid back and not too intense. This recipe works well for fourth-year students on the verge of finishing medical school.

One wouldn't think senioritis would affect students on the threshold of becoming medical doctors, but it happened to most of us. The match was only weeks away and most of us were more concerned with where we would spend the next few years of our lives. However, it never hurts to focus on an often-neglected set of physical exam skills for a month prior to becoming an intern.

My first stroke patient was an elderly male with complete blindness. His caregivers had noticed he was talking funny and was not able to move his facial muscles. After admitting him, we did a thorough history and physical with the help of the patient's daughter. The exact location of a stroke can often be ascertained from the history and physical without imaging.On this patient, the signs had dissipated and imaging was necessary. A CT scan of the head is usually performed right in the ER to rule out a bleed in the brain. CT scans are quick and easy but give less clarity and definition than an MRI. Each has advantages and disadvantages. An acute bleed shows up better on a CT scan giving it the ultimate priority. No acute bleed or midline shift of the brain was discovered.

An MRI of the head was next, along with an MRA to focus on the blood vessels in his brain. Although the MRI uses magnetism and spares the patient the radiation hit that a CT scan produces, it is slower and often creates a long wait for patients. In the meantime, we started him on aspirin to thin his blood and prevent future strokes. To be completely thorough, he was also started on lipid and cholesterol lowering agents.

The vast majority of strokes are caused by plaque build-up over years in patients with high cholesterol. A poor diet and smoking contributes to the process, as well as genetics. An acute event is not caused by complete occlusion of an artery from plaque in most cases. Generally, the plaque ruptures and a blood clot finishes off the artery. This is why a blood thinner is so important in the prevention of strokes and heart attacks.

Over the next couple of days, all of the tests came back negative. The most likely diagnosis was a transient ischemic attack, or TIA, a potential stroke that was all set to occur but didn't. I followed him each morning and performed a neurological exam before the attending arrived to monitor for any recurrences. He was a very pleasant man upon admission, acting very courteous and thankful for our help.

One morning, however, his demeanor changed quite drastically when I asked him some questions to check for his alertness and mental status. He answered poorly on all of the questions and became quite angry at me for bothering him. Although I was taken aback by this change, I knew he had a baseline of moderate dementia, so I thought about ignoring it. Something didn't seem quite right so I left to ask the nurse about his mental status overnight.

For some reason, when I asked if he had been showing any signs of delirium, his nurse and the others standing around actually laughed out loud, another prime example of how medical students aren't taken seriously in the current medical system. I finally got the answer I was waiting for: he was acting completely normal earlier in the morning when she checked on him. I decided to leave and let the residents know my observations. In the meantime, I ran into my classmates and ran the situation by them. At the least, he was having a hospital-induced delirium that the elderly commonly get when transferred from their home environment. At the worst, he could be stroking out. When

I ran the situation by the resident to get his opinion, he downplayed my concerns as well. At that very moment, a nurse interrupted our conversation to let the resident know that this same patient was completely belligerent and peeing all over the floor. "I definitely believe you now," he said, as we all rushed to the room to join the resident already there. He was screaming at everyone that he needed "to get to Loyola."

"You're already at Loyola," the nurse said repeatedly. The fog didn't lift, however, and he kept screaming that he needed to get to Loyola. At that moment, his daughter arrived and helped us alleviate his anxiety. Believing that too many voices and noises were confusing this blind man, the resident sent most of us out of the room, which calmed him down nicely, along with some medication. I learned that an acute mental status change such as this is not typical of a stroke. Strokes are more commonly manifested by motor and sensory deficits similar to what he was admitted for, while delirium manifests as acute mental status changes from a new environment or medication.

Later in the day the nurse I had originally approached acknowledged the fact that she should have listened to me more closely. It was a good feeling to pick up on a deteriorating patient before anyone else. We monitored him for a few days and discharged him to a rehabilitation facility.

For most stroke patients we immediately look at the heart and the carotid arteries in the neck as possible etiologies. Plaques can break off from these locations and embolize to the brain. This patient's carotids were full of plaque and the likely source of his TIA. We determined that he was too elderly and sick to tolerate surgery to clean out his carotids. My other patient at the time, however, was selected for a carotid endarterectomy. My surgical interests caused me to want to follow her to the OR, but, in the end, I decided to leave it to the third-year medical students. I had already had my vascular surgery rotation.

The most common procedure performed on the neurology service is the lumbar puncture, or spinal tap. Although I assisted on one during my emergency month, this was my first chance to perform one myself. My last patient on the wards service was a middle-aged woman with leukemia who had presented with headache and right arm weakness. We had to rule out involvement of the cancer cells in the central nervous system. After laying her on her side, we palpated her lower back to find a good location. She wasn't too overweight, so it was easier than the obese patient in the ER.

The backbone has spinal processes that angle down off the back of each vertebral bone. To get good exposure to the cerebrospinal fluid, one simply pierces the skin in the lower back between the spinal processes, angling the needle slightly upward toward the belly button. The patient lets us know if we hit bone. At first I was afraid I would hurt her, so I was too gentle. I felt resistance on my first pass with the large needle and stopped, fearing I had hit bone but soon realizing it was only ligament. I pushed harder, forcing the needle into her back about three inches, still producing no fluid. As I pressed on, she began to feel the pain and moaned with every movement. I felt bone this time and pulled my needle out, angling it slightly lower towards the feet, still an unsuccessful attempt.

As I angled upward, I popped through some tough resistance and thought I finally had it. When no fluid presented, the resident took over, extracting fluid in about five seconds. If she hadn't intervened, I would have performed my first successful spinal tap. We attached a long tube to the needle and angled it straight up. The clear fluid that bathes the brain and spinal cord slowly began to fill the tube like a thermometer. We measured the opening pressure this way to rule out any serious pathology that may have caused elevated pressure in the brain. Four vials were filled with the CSF and sent to pathology for analysis.

Although it was painful for the patient, she was quite relieved we got it so quickly. She had one earlier at an outside hospital, and it took over an hour to get CSF. We were finished in less than fifteen minutes. Not bad for a novice. In the process of pulling the needle and cleaning up the mess, I spilled CSF fluid on my hands. It was one of those surreal moments in medical school when I stopped thinking about the procedure for a moment to take in the reality of the situation. The clear fluid that had bathed this woman's brain moments prior was now on my gloved hands. No cause could ever be discerned from our testing; consequently, the attendings grew suspicious that her symptoms were either made up or had a psychiatric origin. The exact description of her complaints couldn't be found in any textbook, and, not surprisingly, the numbness conveniently disappeared the following day.

Before I finished my wards rotation, I witnessed two devastating strokes. One was in a 45-year-old gentleman whose carotid neck arteries had dissected for unknown reasons, causing a large stroke in his brain due to lack of blood flow. While he was able to communicate and move his arms the first day, his CT scan the following day showed midline shift of his brain. The stroke was enlarging due to edema and began to smash his brain to the opposite side. Neurosurgery was consulted and took him for immediate surgery where they removed his skull on that side to relieve pressure. The skull was left open for a few days to allow the swelling to resolve; still, he had a very poor prognosis.

The other guy was an elderly man admitted to the hospital for cardiac bypass, stroking the following morning after his surgery. He continued a downward spiral throughout the week. After coding, he was intubated to protect his airway and was successfully resuscitated. The daughters weren't coping with the situation well, so we spent a significant portion of our rounds on a Saturday morning talking to them. After he was stabilized, I was sent home early.

The following Monday I switched to the consult service. It was very similar to the wards service except for more rapid turnover of patients. If any other specialties in the hospital had a neurological question regarding their patient, they would call us. I had never been on a consult service before, so I had to learn some of the etiquette. Instead of a thorough assessment and plan at the end of each daily note, I had only to list the recommendations from a neurological standpoint. I didn't have to manage the myriad of diseases each patient had since that was the role of the primary service. I enjoyed this new-found practice very much. I enjoyed jumping in, giving recommendations, and jumping back out to leave management to the primary service. Perhaps that is why I chose to become a specialist. I enjoy being the master of a small subset of medicine, leaving the rigor of managing diabetes, hypertension, and cardiac disease to others.

The biggest surprise on consults was that no orders could be put in on a patient. Our recommended medications or procedures were accepted, rejected, or completely ignored by the primary team. Recommending better control of a disease outside of the realm of neurology, like diabetes, was also taboo as this would be stepping on the toes of the primary service. After I learned the etiquette of a consulting specialist, I set out to finish my rotation in neurology.

My first patient was a critically ill patient on the cardiothoracic service. She had been transferred from an outside hospital for emergent heart surgery. As they initiated anesthesia, she coded for nearly twenty minutes, responding to resuscitation but remaining mostly unresponsive. I had my first possible brain-dead patient to evaluate. Strict protocol must be followed before declaring a patient completely brain-dead. For one thing, the cerebral hemispheres could be dead, but the brain stem still viable. Can this still be called brain death? Often, primitive reflexes will be maintained in patients with devastating hypoxic brain injuries, leading families to believe their loved one still has hope. Understandably, withdrawing life-sustaining support from a loved one would be difficult when an eye can blink or a foot can move. A good example of this happened to one of my classmates.

In a similarly brain-damaged patient, the foot pulled upward in response to stroking with a reflex hammer, inflating the daughters' hopeful enthusiasm. Unfortunately, my classmate had to explain to them that it was a reflex and a sign of higher-level brain damage.

Right before I entered the room for my first patient, I tried to recall my physical exam lectures in the first two years of medical school. "How do I examine an intubated, unresponsive patient on a ventilator?" I thought to myself. After asking some advice from the residents, I went to the ICU where she was located. I started from the head and worked my way down. With my gloved hands, I pulled open her eyelids and checked her pupils' response to light. They were sluggish, but I observed some movement. At the same time I felt good muscle tone in her eyelids, indicating an intact bilateral facial nerve. As I gently brushed her eyes with some sterile gauze, she blinked from the irritation, proving that two of her cranial nerves were intact, one for receiving the sensation and another for blinking her eyes. I moved farther down to check nerves originating from a lower section of the brainstem. Suctioning down her throat produced an intact gag reflex. I was somewhat optimistic at this point, knowing with certainty that her brainstem was intact. A quick check of the ventilator logs showed she was taking spontaneous breaths over the ventilator, all of which were good signs.

My optimism began to fade as I examined her body. No reflexes could be elicited anywhere in her body. While I pinched her as hard as I could on all four extremities, she made no attempt to pull away. I put pressure on her fingernail-beds with the metal rod of my reflex hammer, an extremely painful procedure to a patient with intact cerebral hemispheres. Again... no response. Even the Babinski sign, the upward pull of the big toe while stroking the bottom of the foot, was absent.

I wrote in my note that day that the brainstem appeared to be intact but cerebral viability was uncertain. After talking with my attending, I recommended an electroencephalogram (EEG) and a cerebral blood flow test. The patient was not very stable, so these tests were slowly completed over the course of the week. Using electrodes over the scalp to monitor for electrical activity, the EEG reported complete silence. In addition, the cerebral blood flow test, with labeled radioactive particles, showed no blood flow to the brain. One by one, the brainstem reflexes I had elicited on day one were disappearing. By the end of the week she was declared brain-dead.

Finding the results very hard to accept, the family kept her on the ventilator a few extra days, eliciting the question of ethics in keeping her on life-support. Unquestionably, this was not a case of persistent vegetative state or coma. This was a dead person being kept alive artificially by machines. The family soon agreed to end it. I paid one last visit to her before everything was withdrawn. "Rest in peace," I said softly, as I touched her arm one last time.

Once a week I had clinic out in Oak Brook with an epilepsy specialist. An interesting relationship between neurology and ENT involving the cranial nerves exists. A seizure patient came to the clinic on my last week that demonstrated this relationship.

The woman had come in for a routine visit, but I noticed right away the asymmetry in her face, the right side of her face showing a distinct droop. As the specialist examined her, he quizzed me on the findings, which, I must admit, totally confused me. I had expected a facial paralysis to be quite simple; and in recognizing my confusion, he walked me through it. When he asked her to smile, the left half of her mouth moved normally while the right half drooped. The curious development was that the previously paralyzed right eye opened. Similarly, when she closed her eyes, the paralyzed right side of the mouth moved.

I was dumbstruck. The patient went on to explain that she had had parotid gland surgery years earlier and her facial nerve had to be cut for the tumor removal. After many months, she began to notice some function return as the nerve began to regenerate and heal. Unfortunately, some of the nerve fibers got crossed in the healing process. Closing her eyes now opened the mouth, and vice versa. Although I never take pleasure in the suffering of a patient, seeing a rare physical exam finding can be quite exhilarating. This was one of those times.

I was still talking about it to the attending later, as he tried to enter the next patient room. I'm sure he appreciated my enthusiasm.

Another prime example of the cross-over between the two specialties was seen in one of our consults. He was a middle-aged man admitted for severe right-sided headache. He also had some numbness around the eye so we were consulted for our opinion. A quick CT scan showed only sinusitis, hence the ENT consultation. By the next day his eye was paralyzed and the pupil dilated. A more detailed examination led us to believe that increased intracranial pressure or brain herniation was unlikely. MRI was quickly ordered which showed an infiltration in the cavernous sinus, a blood-filled cavity behind the eyes in which many important nerves traverse. The leading hypothesis was an invasive fungal sinusitis boring its way through the cavernous sinus.

In the process, the oculomotor nerve was damaged. If this was truly the case, the invasive fungus was only millimeters away from brain. The ENTs took him for immediate surgery to drain the sinuses. A frozen section taken during the procedure confirmed our suspicions: invasive aspergillosis. He was started on IV antifungals and monitored closely.

As in most rotations, I personally followed many patients but had a couple of long-term patients the entire time. One was the brain dead patient I have described; the other was a burn patient that stroked after surgery to clean the wounds. The massive stroke was on the left side of her brain, likely eliminating any chance she would ever talk again. I performed the same set of physical exam steps on her as I did on the brain dead patient. Only with her, she grimaced with pain every time I pinched her or put pressure on her nail beds. Each day I would apologize profusely, explaining the need to check the function of her nerves for further damage caused by the stroke.

The burn unit on the seventh floor of the hospital also required specific protocol. Absolutely no food or drinks were allowed. Just left of the entrance, a quick left was taken to remove the white coat, a common transport vehicle of antibiotic-resistant pathogens. Hands were washed and a gown, face mask, and gloves adorned.

After an acute insult in the brain, edema and swelling can continue to cause damage for nearly a week, three to five being the peak. We finally persuaded the primary burn team unit to start her on Mannitol, a diuretic that decreases intracranial pressure in patients such as this. Their only hesitation was that fluid balance in a burn patient is extremely difficult. Fluids are lost at dramatic rates when the skin is not intact, generally necessitating large amounts of IV fluids. Giving Mannitol was going in the opposite direction. A careful algorithm was put in place; and after a week, she stabilized and was transferred to a long-term care facility. A long, difficult road of rehabilitation was in store for her, but at least she escaped with her life.

Neurology was an interesting rotation. I was glad to brush up on my neurological skills but even happier to have the last required rotation of fourth year over. The last week of the rotation was cut short due to match week. The match is the process wherein medical students find a residency at which to train. I will describe the match with an ENT perspective, but it basically is the same for everyone.

In the summer of my fourth year, I began the application process through an on-line web site called ERAS. The entire application including letters of recommendation, extracurricular activities, leadership experiences, grades, and boards scores are loaded onto ERAS to be dispersed electronically to any residency of choice.

All of this activity happened concurrently with my fourth-year rotations as I auditioned at another school, studied for Step 2 of the boards, and readied myself for intern year. After ERAS is completed, applications are sent to the residencies who then judge one's fate. Because otolaryngology is an extremely competitive field, I applied to many different places around the country, centering on the Midwest but also applying elsewhere to increase my chances of matching. The more schools applied to, however, the more the price goes up. Add this onto the cost of flying around to interview, and the financial strain becomes intense.

Not coming from a wealthy family necessitated medical school loans, which basically paid for everything, including the cost of living. Since interviewing and things of that nature were not included in the loan money, my wife and I went into a lot of credit card debt my senior year, which we hoped would be paid off during my residency.

I concentrated most of my interviews in December since I took that month off from school. It worked out nicely since I had the week of Thanksgiving and Christmas off as well. This time was also used to study for Step 2 of the boards. I sat in the coffee shops for hours every day, dividing my time between rapid studying and interviews. My poor wife had erroneously thought she would see me much more than she did, considering it was vacation. However, she understood what I was trying to accomplish.

I was pleased overall with the number of interviews I received from residencies, but I still couldn't hide my nervousness. Once one gets to the interview, every applicant is pretty much on the same playing field. They take into consideration the entire package of grades, board scores, and personality.

The interview process introduced me to sights of intrigue and impressive facilities. Seeing different institutions actually made the ranking of schools more difficult, of where to rank whom, especially since all of my places of interview proved to be exceptional. Some had certain strengths that others didn't, such as more expensive facilities and learning tools. On my tour at one famous institution, we walked into a lab room where one of the residents was operating on a human head. "All you have to do is call the lab the day before and they'll have a head thawed and waiting for you," she said. I was awestruck. Any time I wanted to learn a new procedure and build my surgical knowledge, I could practice on an expensive human cadaver head. Even after gross anatomy, seeing a head on a platter was quite an experience. That was perhaps my most memorable moment of all of my interviews.

Early in the second semester of fourth year, students and residencies around the country begin the difficult process of formulating the rank list into a computer system. A lot of energy goes into placing them into their desired position on the final list. This was very difficult, since I had to carefully consider the advantages as well as the repercussions for not only myself but also for my wife.

I finally made my decision, submitting my rank list once and for all. Each student and residency across the country did likewise. In March, a computer placed us into the appropriate slot, and our fate for the next few years was sealed.

On Monday of match week, an email is sent out informing everyone whether or not he or she matched. In the event that a student doesn't match, which does happen occasionally, the scramble takes place. On Tuesday every unmatched student sits in a single room with the deans. Copies of resumes are ready and waiting to fax to any open positions around the country. Generally a few spots in each specialty remain which, for some reason, do not fill. Because every unmatched student is desperate to slide into a spot, he or she may have to make a split-second decision over the phone to take a position and move family across the country to a hospital that is not even familiar.

Within a day or two, the scramble is over and most students find a spot in either their specialty of choice or a general internship year.

Unfortunately, a few students don't match at all. A year of their life is lost. In a career choice that takes many years to train, this is no insignificant matter. Many perform research in the field of their choice or a general internship. Some have to consider changing their career plans to a specialty that is less competitive than the specialty they love. It's not a good situation, and I hoped that I would not have to go through it.

The culmination of four years of medical school was coming to a peak. A buzz was in the air unlike any I had experienced in medical school. The excitement permeated every discussion, both in the hospital and outside with my family. On Monday of match week, I excused myself from rounds, my stomach in knots. After making my way to the fourth floor computer lab of the school, I called my wife. She was at work in downtown Chicago and far more nervous than I. I had her check my email while I checked the match website. Consequently, my wife knew the news before I did. Good news: I had matched! No other information was given, so we had to wait until Thursday to find out the location. A relief poured over me that I hadn't felt in over half a year. Unfortunately, a couple other classmates applying to ENT weren't so lucky. They would have to reapply the following year.

Thursday came around quickly and everyone gathered at 10 AM in the atrium of the medical school. My wife joined me while we nervously talked with classmates and their families. The balconies above were lined with younger students looking down on us with amazement, something I had done in previous years. I smiled at the memories of looking down at the seniors, jealous that my time had not yet come. Time had flown so quickly.

At 10:50 AM the Dean of the Medical School gave a brief speech, followed by the associate deans. Tables covered with white envelopes lined the perimeter. All students had one with their name on it. At 11 AM, on March 20th, 2008 the announcement was made to open the envelopes. Having already migrated next to my table, I quickly grabbed the envelope, running with Nicole around the corner to experience the revelation in private. She held on tightly as I opened it.

Henry Ford Hospital in Detroit, Michigan.

We were ecstatic! We had aimed for a Midwestern city, and I had loved the hospital during my interview. The long wait was finally over. The next five years of my life were already set in motion. The match is a legally binding contract and cannot be undone except under extreme circumstances. That night we celebrated and made plans for the next chapter in our lives. Only one elective was left, and I felt as if I already had one foot out the door. I spent some of my free time tying up loose ends that were needed for graduation. Things were happening very quickly now.

Chapter 19: Neuroradiology

My reasons for choosing my last elective in neuroradiology came from a desire to brush up on head and neck anatomy and imaging prior to beginning a residency in otolaryngology. Surprisingly, I had much more patient contact than I had originally thought. I had envisioned sitting in a dark room all day reading films. I spent most mornings with my physician performing procedures. Neuroradiologists perform a fellowship after a five-year radiology residency to become a subspecialist. They not only focus on the head and neck but also the spine.

My first morning was spent in the reading room. I entered a dark room full of computers and large monitors. Each attending had a computer and was silently reading films. I joined a guy I had heard was more open to teaching students. Before him were five large computer monitors and a keyboard. He used the monitor on the right as his computer to pull patient charts and write his reports. The other four monitors were further subdivided into two to nine smaller screens each with a specific cut of anatomy. When an MRI was brought up for a specific patient, each screen filled with a different cut. He often linked them together so that each image would move in sequence as he scrolled with his mouse. I was disappointed to find that the vast majority of films were non-ENT related. I began to fear that choosing this elective was a mistake.

The following morning I joined the rotation coordinator for some procedures. He was a great mentor and one of the nicest attendings I had the privilege of working with. Most of the procedures we performed were cerebral angiograms. After covering ourselves with lead vests, we gave the patient a mild sedative to take off the edge. After a small incision was made in the groin, my attending introduced a catheter into the femoral artery, maneuvering the catheter tip under fluoroscopic guidance to the vessels in the neck.

Dye would be injected at specific times to study the cerebral vasculature. Stroke and aneurysm patients are primary candidates for a cerebral angiogram. When the intervention was for diagnostic purposes only, the day went very quickly. However, a couple of patients with aneurysms needed to be treated.

My first aneurysm patient was a woman in her fifties who smiled to hide her nervousness. We gave her the usual words of affirmation that "everything was going to be fine." Using dye, we quickly spotted the aneurysm. The physician inserted a tiny wire through the catheter and worked it all the way up to the brain. I watched on the monitor as the wire was inserted into the small, aneurysmal sac. The wire began to coil on itself until the sac was completely obliterated. Over time it would completely embed into the wall and eliminate any risk of rupture and death. We pulled the catheter out and began to wake the patient as she was put completely under for this particular case. She was still rather groggy, but the attending wanted to do a quick neurological exam to rule out any complications. She complied with his commands by moving all extremities.

Satisfied with the response, the attending left the room to begin his dictation. I decided to make myself helpful on this rotation and aided in cleaning the room. The technicians later commented that they had never seen a medical student help out so much with the menial tasks of patient care. I bagged up the trash bags and carried them out of the room, anxious to get the room ready for the next patient. The dumpster was in the back room, so I had to walk through another specials lab to get to it.

Pausing at the door, I saw a patient in the room awaiting her procedure. The technicians told me to go ahead and pass since the sterile tray hadn't been opened yet. As I walked past the patient, I saw that she stared up at the ceiling with obvious nervousness. I had no idea at the time that she would be dead in half an hour.

When I got back to my room, the anesthesiologists were still trying to wake the aneurysm patient. My attending came back into the room to do another neuro exam.

"Ma'am, can you open your eyes?" the attending said.

No response.

"Ma'am!" he shouted.

No response.

He reached over to her shoulder and pinched her as hard as he could, his voice elevating dramatically.

"WAKE UP!" he shouted as he ripped off her oxygen mask and began smacking her in the face.

"This isn't normal," he said. The anesthesiologist agreed.

"INDUCE HER! WE'RE GOING BACK IN!"

The room went into a flurry of activity as they prepared to get into her vasculature. I helped as well I could, injecting heparin into saline bags for the procedure. The attending moved faster than I had ever seen him move. We called for neurosurgery in case emergency surgery would be needed. When dye was finally injected in the brain, a large clot could be seen adjacent to the coil. The dye-filled portion of the artery had narrowed right behind the coil, signifying that the vessel lumen was full of clot. We began blasting her with clot-busting medicines in the artery, extremely dangerous medicines that can easily cause hemorrhaging in the brain. Hour after hour we fought to save her from stroking out and dying, recording each clot buster dose as we were quickly approached the danger level.

It is bizarre how major events always seem to happen at once in the hospital. Right across the wall from our room, the code began on the patient I had seen on my garbage run. Both rooms were now in a panic to save their patients. It was not a good day for the specials lab. Unfortunately, the other patient was not as fortunate as ours.

When the clot in our patient finally dissipated, we began the process of waking her, the attending anxious to do a neuro exam to see if she had any function left. Damage to her brain would be evident as soon as she awoke. We were lucky. She seemed to have recovered completely. We transported her to the Neuro ICU and explained to her that she had developed a clot, moving into an immediate coma. She sounded surprised and couldn't remember anything.

I was asked to keep a close eye on her. During one of my neuro exams later in the afternoon, I noticed that her left eye wouldn't move to the right. I reported my finding to the ICU resident, fearful that a bleed may be developing. The problem resolved over a few hours, but everyone commended me on my find, my attending bragging about my performance for the next two days. I didn't mind the attention.

Another interesting procedure I witnessed was a kyphoplasty. Elderly patients with osteoarthritis can develop painful compression fractures of their vertebral bodies. The neuroradiologists can treat their fractures under fluoroscopic guidance and provide them with immediate pain relief. The patients are placed on the same interventional table with their back exposed so that the crushed vertebral body can be found and marked for easy access.

After the area is prepped and anesthetized with local, a small incision is made a couple of centimeters off the midline. Next, a trochar is carefully pressed into the backbone through the tiny incision, guided by fluoroscopy to spare the spinal cord and prevent complete paralysis. The trochar is then screwed into the bone and retracted. A balloon catheter is inserted into the newly created cavity and opened up to expand the cavity. Finally, injected liquid cement immediately hardens to support the severely fractured bone. The patients I witnessed had immediate relief from their pain. It has to be a very rewarding procedure to perform.

Most of my free time was spent preparing a large presentation for my last day of the rotation. I picked a topic that related to my field of interest and put a lot of effort into it. When the last day approached, I wasn't even nervous about my presentation; instead, I was giddy about finishing my last day of medical school. We did a cerebral angiogram just prior to my lecture. However, just as we were about to leave we got a call from the Emergency Department. They had an unresponsive woman with a large bleed in her brain. She needed an angiogram to see if anything was salvageable. I quickly gave my presentation to the radiology residents and other medical students and rushed back to the specials lab. The patient was already on the table being prepared for the procedure. The entire neurosurgery team was there as well, and tensions were high. The angiogram was performed and the bleed identified. Before we could talk about how to treat the bleed, her blood pressure skyrocketed into the 300s. The monitor that neurosurgery had inserted into her skull began to fill with blood, signifying she had blown her ventricles with a new bleed.

The prognosis at this point was extremely grave. We continued to treat her while talks began with the family to make her DNR. After stabilization, we aborted any angiographic treatment and transported her to the ICU where she would die. It saddened me that my last patient of medical school wasn't going to make it, somewhat dampening the celebration I had planned. After meeting with my attending one last time, I walked out of Loyola for the last time as a medical student. Spring had come and the weather was beautiful for what seemed like the first time that year. I called Nicole and my immediate family on the ride home to share my exhilaration. The marathon was finally over.

Chapter 20: Graduation: The Beginning

First described by Hippocrates, the father of medicine, *Facies Hippocratica* is a term used to describe the characteristic appearance on a patient's face just before death. After having gone through my years of training, I know this look quite well, still seeing the face of every patient I lost during that time. These enduring images constantly remind me of my desire to become a doctor: to improve the quality of life and to strive to save life. These same images remind me of the purpose behind this book: to remember those patients I lost during this phase of an incredible journey. I don't want to forget those who touched my life and shaped me into the doctor I am today and will be tomorrow. I want you to remember them as well. It is my hope that the readers of this book will reflect upon the lives of those who lived and died in the halls of Loyola Hospital.

Not long after I walked out of Loyola for the last time, my family and I gathered at Navy Pier in downtown Chicago for graduation. Four years of medical school had gone by so quickly, yet the walk across the stage to receive my diploma slowed to a surreal realization that my life's work had just begun. Although part of me worried that I was not fully prepared to bear the title of *physician*, I was confident in the doctors at Loyola who had had enough faith in us, investing the time and effort necessary to produce quality doctors. The future looked bright as I anticipated a life's work dedicated to helping the sick and saving lives. I tried not to be too proud in my new title of M.D., but admittedly, I was beaming with pride. I felt as if I had become a member of an exclusive club, the initiation comprised of years of sacrifice and hard work.

Year after year, throughout the centuries, graduating classes of medical schools around the world have recited a pledge, swearing an oath to protect the ones we serve. While each nation and class have their own version of the creed, the promise to strive to preserve life and the promise not to abuse the privileges given to us remain the same.

My official certification came when I recited Loyola's version of the Hippocratic Oath. While the ancient physicians swore by the Greek gods, I recited my vow by Jesus Christ, promising to protect and uphold the liberties given to us by God, to fight for life, and to be an advocate for the sick and afflicted. I swore to sacrifice sleep and personal time with my family to dedicate myself to the most wonderful calling I have ever known. I know I will never forget my years of training, never presuming to think I am perfect, but instead, remembering my calling as a mission to serve those in need.

As I write this last chapter, I am a matter of weeks into my surgical internship where the stress is a completely new ballgame. Having the responsibility of taking care of someone during a fragile phase of life when death is possible is an overwhelming task, but this is what I want to do. The awesome burden of sometimes being the only doctor in the hospital for more than fifty patients reminds me of my mission. This is what I want to do. While this memoir is meant to tell the story of an American medical student, it is much more than that. It is meant to describe the sacred bond of the doctor-patient relationship, and to show that a doctor has an obligation to the patients who put all trust in him or her. This is the mission I speak of and the motto I will live by: "For I was ill and you cared for me."

Printed in Great Britain
by Amazon.co.uk, Ltd.,
Marston Gate.